The Unplanned Pregnancy Book for Teens and College Students

1/12

The Unplanned Pregnancy Book
for Teens and College Students

By Dorrie Williams-Wheeler

Portions of this book have been adapted with permission from *The Unplanned
Pregnancy Handbook-Real Life Stories, Resources and Information to Help You*
which was written by Dorrie Williams-Wheeler © 2003.

Library of Congress Cataloging-in-Publication Data
ISBN 0-9747832-3-4
Published By
Sparkledoll Productions
PO Box 56173
Virginia Beach, VA 23456
http://www.sparkledoll.com

cover design-Sparkledoll Productions

Sparkledoll Productions publishes books for teens and college age students.
View our complete list of titles at www.sparkledoll.com.

Disclaimer- The information in this book should not be substituted for advice
from an actual physician. This book is only meant to provide information and
guidance. The author is an educator and makes no claims that she is a medical
physician or licensed counselor. This book also features real life stories from
young women who have been faced with unplanned pregnancies. Names and
locations were changed. Stories were also edited for clarity and space. The
participants signed releases to have their stories used for the book. Any
similarity to any person living or dead is pure coincidence.

First printing

Acknowledgements

I would like to thank all of the women who shared their stories with me to make this book possible. Whether they met with me in person or shared their stories via fax, phone or e-mail this book would not have been possible without them. When I put the word out that I was looking for young women who wanted to share stories of unplanned pregnancies, the response was truly overwhelming. I thank all of you and wish I would have had the space to accommodate all of the stories I received and was told.

I would like to thank all of the facilities and centers who gave me insight into their operations—the doctors offices, the state run organizations, the university family housing departments, the maternity shelters, everyone. I would like to thank all of the maternity shelters employees who took the time to let me tour their facilities and who also provided me insight as to the services they provide. Also, I want to thank all of the people who put up with my thousands of questions about the various topics covered in this book.

Be sure to visit The Unplanned Pregnancy Book for Teens and College Students on the web at www.unplannedpregnancybook.com.

Table of Contents

Foreword
Chapter 1-You Think You're Pregnant..................................1
Chapter 2- Get Ready...You're Going To Be A Mommy!.........6
Chapter 3-Baby Gear...What To Buy and What Can Wait........32
Chapter 4- Continuing Your Education & Parenting...............38
Chapter 5- Everything You Ever Wanted To Know About DNA Paternity Testing...47
Chapter 6- Abortion-Answers to Your Questions..................55
Chapter 7-Adoption-The Option....................................71
Chapter 8- Desperate Acts-Safe Haven Laws......................80
Chapter 9- Birth Control For The Future...........................85
Chapter 10- Web Resources..90
Chapter 11- Phone Numbers.. 101
Chapter 12- Related Reading..104
Discussion Questions, Exercises and Activities...................108
About The Author..111
References..112

Foreword

Okay, you're pregnant and this is not how you planned things. It was a surprise, an accident, an unexpected event and you just don't know what to do.

How will I tell my parents?
What if I don't have insurance?
If I have a baby can I still go to college?
What should I do????????

The Unplanned Pregnancy Book for Teens and College Students is a helpful guide written to provide you with information and resources that can help you come to terms with how to handle your unplanned pregnancy. This book is not written to influence or change your mind about how you should deal with your pregnancy. This book aims to be an educational guide that you can refer to again and again as a resource.

Throughout the book you will find stories from young women who have faced unplanned pregnancy. These women shared their stories in hopes that you readers will learn from their experiences. All of the stories are true. Only the names and locations were changed. Stories were edited for clarity and length. The information in this book should not be substituted for advice from an actual physician. This book was written to be a guide in your quest for knowledge, not a substitute for actual advice from a doctor or psychologist.

Hopefully, by the time that you are finished reading this book you will have a plan as to how you are going to deal with your unplanned pregnancy. If you found this book to be a helpful resource, please consider passing it on to someone you think might need it.

Educate yourself.
Make a plan.
Take action!

CHAPTER 1-You Think You're Pregnant

DETERMINING THAT YOU ARE PREGNANT

If you think you are pregnant, the first thing that you need to do is to confirm this information as soon as possible. The first sign of a possible pregnancy for many women is a late period. However, some teens and young women have irregular periods, so just because your period is late or doesn't come at all this isn't a sure sign that you are pregnant. Another sign of early pregnancy is nausea and vomiting. Some women may feel tenderness in their breasts. Although these early symptoms may indicate pregnancy, just because you may experience one, none, or all of these symptoms, it is still important to take a pregnancy test.

If you suspect that you may be pregnant, you can purchase a home pregnancy test from your local drug store. Home pregnancy tests range in price from $7-$18 dollars. Home pregnancy tests look for a hormone named hCG in your urine. The presence of hCG is a strong indication of pregnancy. This hormone is produced by the placenta when a woman is pregnant. The hCG hormone can be detected in blood and urine as early as six days after fertilization has taken place.

If you are a minor, you don't need your parents permission to purchase a home pregnancy test. Some stores keep pregnancy tests in locked glass cases. Technically, a store cannot refuse to sell you a test because of your age. If a store refuses to sell you a test, alert the manager or else go to another store. The test can be taken in the privacy of your home. Many women prefer to take a home pregnancy test to confirm their pregnancy before they actually go see a doctor.

Some tests can be taken as early as a few days before your period is actually late. However, the tests are more accurate when performed close to the actual date of your period or shortly after your period is late.

If you do not feel comfortable administering the test to yourself, because you feel you may do the test wrong or for other reasons, there are many facilities that offer confidential pregnancy testing.

OKAY YOU'RE PREGNANT, WHAT'S NEXT?

Pregnancy lasts approximately 280 days, which is a little over nine months. If you find out that you are pregnant 4 weeks after your last menstrual cycle, you are already considered to be 4 weeks pregnant.

It is important to find out just how pregnant that you are for several reasons. If you are planning on continuing your pregnancy, you will need to make arrangements to see a doctor for pre-natal care. If this pregnancy was unplanned you may not have the necessary insurance for prenatal care and you may need to make arrangements to obtain medical insurance. Now is also the time to begin saving money if you plan to become a parent. Also, if you are considering adoption, now is the time to begin investigating the type of adoption that you feel is best for you.

If you are considering terminating your pregnancy you need to plan accordingly. First trimester abortions are most common and have the least complications. They are also far less expensive than second trimester abortions. Therefore, if you are planning to have an abortion, you will need to find out how far along you are in your pregnancy. After you determine how far along you are in your pregnancy, you will need to find an abortion provider in your area. Once you find an abortion provider you will need to find out how much the procedure will cost.

Think hard about your options. You may decide to seek counseling before you actually decide how you are going to proceed. You may wish to discuss this information with your parents or boyfriend. Take time to think about your unplanned pregnancy, but don't take too much time. Time is of the essence and the sooner you make your decision the sooner you can proceed with your course of action.

2

WHO TO TELL AND HOW TO TELL THEM

BOYFRIEND/CHILD'S FATHER

Your boyfriend may be the first person you tell. If this pregnancy was unplanned the news may come as a shock to him. If you all have a close relationship he may be your rock in dealing with this shocking news. If your first sign that you might be pregnant is a missed period, you may want to tell him that you suspect that you are pregnant. You all then as a couple can make a plan to have a pregnancy test performed. If you are pregnant, as a couple you all can determine how you will proceed with the unplanned pregnancy. As a couple you all can work on a plan as to how you want to tell both sets of parents. If both you and your boyfriend are over the age of 18 and living on your own, you may not need to share the information with parents right away, or at all depending on your course of action.

If your pregnancy resulted from a casual relationship or a relationship that is already over, telling him might not be an easy thing. If the relationship was strained you may want to consult with parents or a friend before discussing the situation with him.

PARENTS

This is not something that you want your parents to find out about through the grapevine. It is best to tell your parents as soon as possible. If you are in a situation where you truly fear your parents, and you worry about your physical safety or feel that they might try to influence you to handle the unplanned pregnancy in a manner you may not want to, think of an alternative adult to confide in. In this situation, you may want to confide in an aunt, counselor or family friend.

An unplanned pregnancy is not something that you want to go through alone—especially if you are a minor. If you are a college student over the age of 18, you are mentally more well equipped to handle this situation than a young woman under the age of 18 who is still living at home with her parents.

How to tell your parents?

Don't beat around the bush. Simply sit down your mother or father and tell them that you think that you are pregnant. You might want to schedule a meeting at a time when you know that your mom or dad or both have time to sit down and talk. This is not the kind of thing that you want to spring on them as they are heading out the door to work or when they are expecting company. This is not going to be an easy conversation to have with your parents. They may not have even known you were sexually active. This conversation may be the most grown up conversation that you will have in your life, but you need your parents to help you with this situation. They can be your support system.

FRIENDS

If your friend is your confidant and you feel that she can help you in this situation you may wish to tell her. Now if your friend is someone who likes to gossip, you might not want to tell her right away. Not that you want to keep this information a secret, it's just that you might not want to tell everyone right away for several reasons. If you have not yet decided what you plan to do about your unplanned pregnancy you don't want everyone to know that you are pregnant. For instance, if you are on the fence about raising the baby yourself or giving it up for adoption, you might not want all of the attention that comes along with people knowing that you are pregnant. Let's just say you don't want the info all around school right away. Additionally, many women wait until their second trimester before they start telling the world that they are expecting.

AUNT/FAMILY FRIEND/NEUTRAL PARTY

If you have a situation where you can't tell your parents, because they are abusive or you feel they won't understand, you may want to tell a neutral party like an aunt or a family friend. This neutral party may be able to help you tell your parents, or if you are truly too scared to tell your parents, they may be able to tell them for you. If you don't want to involve your parents in your unplanned pregnancy because you are older or in college, a neutral party may be someone that you can confide in and that will help you make plans as to how to deal with your unplanned pregnancy.

CHAPTER 2- Get Ready...You're Going To Be A Mommy!

This pregnancy thing took you by surprise but you have decided that you are going to hang in there and see this thing through and become a parent. There is a lot of planning and work involved with becoming a new parent, so enjoy any rest you can get now.

SEEING A DOCTOR
Once you suspect that you may be pregnant, it is a good idea to schedule an appointment to see a doctor. If you do not have an obstetrician/gynecologist, you can schedule your initial visit with your family doctor or a general practitioner. The doctor will then confirm your pregnancy and refer you to an OB/GYN for prenatal care. Confirming your pregnancy is important, because although rare, sometimes home pregnancy tests can be wrong. Many women fear they may be pregnant because their period has stopped or is late, and often pregnancy is not the cause for this problem.

PRENATAL CARE
If you have decided to continue your pregnancy to term, prenatal care is vital for both you and your baby. If you do not have insurance, there are programs that will assist you in obtaining insurance and/or free or reduced prenatal care.

During your first and second trimester you will visit your doctor once a month for prenatal care. Starting at 30 weeks, during your third trimester you may begin seeing your doctor every two weeks. During your ninth month starting at 36 weeks you may begin seeing your doctor once a week. If your pregnancy is considered high risk you may see your doctor more often through out the duration of your pregnancy.

Prenatal care consists of monitoring and testing you and the baby. During the first visit you will be asked about previous pregnancies, whether you smoke, drink or take any drugs, and about the family medical history of you and your partner. During routine visits you will be subject to various tests. At most routine visits you will be weighed, given a urine screening, and have your blood pressure taken. Your doctor will listen to fetal heart tones with a Doppler, and may ask you general questions about your health.

The following pages include tests that you may be given during your prenatal care. Please keep in mind that every prenatal care facility is different and you may not be given all of the tests mentioned. Your doctor will make sure that you get the best prenatal care that you need to have a happy and healthy pregnancy. Also, depending on your age and the nature of your pregnancy your doctor may schedule additional tests not listed below.

FIRST TRIMESTER TESTS

Pregnancy Test-You will be given a pregnancy test even if you took an over the counter test. The doctor must confirm your pregnancy.

Urine Test-The urine test looks for sugar and protein in your urine. Too much sugar can mean that your body is not processing sugar properly and protein in the urine can signal high blood pressure or a kidney problem. The urine test can also detect bladder infections and other urinary tract infections. This important screening can find out many things.

Blood Test-At your first visit blood will be drawn. The blood tests determine your blood type and detect anemia and any infections the mother may have. The blood drawn may also be used for various screening exams, such as to see if the mother is a carrier for Sickle Cell Anemia. Your Rh type will also be determined. Rh type refers to the presence of positive or absence of negative Rh factor in your blood. Your Rh type is noted to look for Rh incompatibility between you and the fetus. Rh incompatibility occurs when a Rh negative mother produces an Rh positive child.

Culture of the Cervix and Vagina- The doctor performs this test to determine if you have certain diseases such as chlamydia, gonorrhea or other sexually transmitted diseases. These tests are important because these diseases can be potentially harmful to the fetus. If the cultures come back positive you will be treated.

Pap Smear- Even if you just had one, your doctor may perform a Pap Smear as part of your routine prenatal care. The Pap Smear tests for cervical cancer.

HIV Test- Some doctors offices give HIV test to pregnant women. Not all prenatal care facilities offer this test. You will be given the opportunity to sign a consent form and you can object to this test if do want the test performed. If your test results are positive, you may be put on special drugs to avoid potentially passing the HIV virus to your child.

SECOND TRIMESTER TESTS

Maternal Serum Alpha-Fetoprotein and Multiple Marker Screening- This test is usually given between 15-18 weeks of pregnancy. This test is performed by drawing a sample of blood. The test checks the levels of Alpha-Fetoprotein. Abnormal levels can indicate Downs Syndrome or Spina Bifida.

Ultrasound-An ultrasound is a test that uses sound waves to produce pictures of the fetus. Some physicians will perform a first trimester ultrasound which is known as a transvaginal ultrasound. A first trimester ultrasound can accurately date the pregnancy. A first trimester pregnancy can also ensure that the pregnancy is proceeding as it should. A second trimester ultrasound is usually given between 18-20 weeks. The second trimester ultrasound is known as the transabdominal ultrasound. It can verify your due date, detect malformations in the fetus, detect multiple pregnancies, or detect other complications, such as a low lying placenta. Another ultrasound may be offered during the third trimester to determine the position of the fetus. Often depending on your insurance plan or doctor, you may only have one ultrasound during your pregnancy or none at all. It really depends on your physician and insurance plan. An ultrasound is not performed in every pregnancy.

There is a new ultrasound technology gaining in popularity among doctors and future mothers. This type of ultrasound is known as the 4D ultrasound. This type of ultrasound can capture 3 dimensional moving images of your baby. This technology is exclusive to GE. With this type of ultrasound you can see images of your fetus that are more clear and baby-like than the other ultrasound methods. 4D ultrasounds are more expensive than the traditional transabdominal ultrasounds so be certain that your insurance will pay for this type of ultrasound if your doctor suggests it.

There are boutique places that will allow you to come into a mall or strip mall to get an ultrasound. These ultrasounds are not medical ultrasounds that look for approximate fetus age, length, deformities, the type of things that your doctor and ultrasound technician look for when you get an ultrasound at your OB/GYN office. These ultrasound boutiques give you pictures and sometimes a video tape of your ultrasound.

Prenatal Peek is a company that offers 4D ultrasounds for entertainment purposes. They offer non diagnostic ultrasounds, meaning just the pictures not a medical screening. They offer 10-30 minute ultrasound sessions. Services that they offer include photographs, videos, a web page, gender determination and more. Prenatal Peek only employs qualified sonographers, but this ultrasound still should not take the place of the ultrasound that your doctor may prescribe.

Your insurance most likely will not pay for this non diagnostic ultrasound.

Additional Information
GE 4D Ultrasound
http://www.gehealthcare.com/rad/us/4d/

Non-medical ultrasounds
http://www.prenatalpeek.com

Amniocentesis- This test looks for birth defects in the fetus. This test is not always given in routine pregnancies in women under the age of 30, so it's not likely that it will be part of your routine pre-natal care. This test may be ordered if a woman has an abnormal Maternal Serum Alpha-Fetoprotein and Multiple Marker screening test result. The test is preformed when the doctor puts a needle into the mothers uterus through her belly and draws amniotic fluid. If you are interested in prenatal DNA paternity screening your doctor may perform an amniocentesis to gather a testing sample.

Glucose Screening-Glucose screening is another blood test. The mother is given a special sugary drink to ingest. Her blood is then drawn about an hour later to test the sugar levels in her blood. This test is usually given between 24-28 weeks.

THIRD TRIMESTER TESTS

Fetal Non-Stress Test
A non-stress test is an external test performed in high risk pregnancies during the third trimester. The test is performed by having the woman lie down and wear two belts. One of the belts monitors for contractions and the other belt monitors the fetal heart beat. The test is performed for various reasons including gestational diabetes, decreased fetal movement, or if a woman has gone beyond her due date.

Group B Strep Test
Many healthy women carry Group B Strep bacteria, however, this bacteria can be harmful to newborns. Between 35-37 weeks the

woman's vagina and rectum is swabbed and tested. If Group B
Strep is present, the woman may be given antibiotics during
delivery to protect the infant.

INSURANCE

Being a pregnant woman you are going to need insurance to cover
your prenatal care and the birth of your child. Without insurance
this type of medical treatment can be very costly. Between exams
and tests your first prenatal visit can cost several hundred dollars.

If you are a minor and on your parents insurance, you should
have your parents contact their insurance company to find out if
they will cover prenatal care for a dependent. You should also find
out if they will be able to add the baby to their insurance after the
birth of the child.

If you are insured through your employment, college, or spouse
it is always a good idea to call your insurance company and inform
them of your pregnancy. Some insurance companies require that
you have a referral to obtain OB/GYN care for prenatal services.
Others do not require this step. It is also a good idea to know
exactly what services are covered for your prenatal care. Whereas
some insurance companies will allow a woman to get numerous
ultrasounds through out her pregnancy and allow every test under
the sun to be performed, other insurance companies may only
cover one ultrasound, whereas some may not pay for an ultrasound
at all unless deemed medically necessary. Every insurance
company is different so it is best that you know the ends and outs
of your insurance company regarding your prenatal care.

Insurance companies only give you a certain amount of time
after the birth of the child for you to enroll the child on to your
insurance policy. Contact the insurance company immediately after
the birth of your child. Your hospital bill for the child birth will be
separate than the babies medical bill, and if the child is not added
on to an insurance plan within a certain time frame you may have
to pay for their portion of the bill.

PROGRAMS TO HELP YOU

You've just discovered that you are pregnant. You may still be in school or not have a job. Depending on your situation you may not have health insurance. The above may or may not apply to you, but no matter how desperate your situation may seem there are many programs out there to help you continue your pregnancy if you desire to. Once you have the knowledge, you can proceed with your pregnancy with greater ease.

MEDICAID

Medicaid is a form of insurance for low income individuals. Medicaid was established under the Federal Social Security Act to allow states to provide medical assistance for individuals on public aid and also for low income individuals. If you have income coming into your household, yet do not have sufficient income for medical insurance, you may qualify for Medicaid assistance. To apply for Medicaid you would contact your local Department of Health and Human Services Office. Some states call their Department of Health and Human Services-Social Services. Medicaid insurance will allow you to obtain necessary prenatal care and it will cover your child birth for you and your child.

FOOD STAMPS

The Food Stamp program is a program sponsored by the US Department of Agriculture. This program provides benefits to low income households. Depending on your state, a food stamp recipient will receive actual food stamp coupons that can be used at grocery stores to purchase food items or they may be issued an EBT card. The EBT, which is short for Electronic Benefits Transfer Card, puts a food stamp recipients benefits on an electronic debit card. Even if you do not qualify for cash benefits or Medicaid, you may still qualify for The Food Stamp Program.

The size of your family and your income will determine how much you will receive in monthly benefits. To apply for Food Stamps contact your local social services or human services department. To find the nearest location in your area, The Food Stamp Program has a 24 hour toll free phone number. This is not a number that you can call to apply by phone for Food Stamp benefits. This number will only tell you where you can apply for Food Stamp benefits in your area. In addition to helping you locate the number to your nearest social services or health department, the hotline also provides pre-recorded nutrition information. The number was established in 1999. The toll-free Food Stamp information number is 1-800-221-5689.

THE WOMEN INFANT & CHILDREN PROGRAM (WIC)
The WIC program is a program developed to help the well being of low income women, infants and children under the age of 5. The WIC program provides nutritious food to women and children. The program also provides mothers with formula for their infants.
Many women are not aware of the WIC program. The WIC program is not as difficult to qualify for as the Food Stamp program. Therefore, if you are turned down for Food Stamps, you may be eligible to receive WIC benefits. It is also possible to qualify for both WIC and Food Stamps. Even a low income married woman and her children can qualify for WIC assistance. A pregnant woman can receive WIC benefits for herself during her pregnancy and for six months after the birth of her child. She can receive WIC benefits for herself for up to one year if she is breast feeding. A child can remain on the WIC program up until the age of 5. WIC serves 45% of the infants born in the United States.

In addition to providing nutritious foods to women and children, the WIC program also provides women with nutrition information, health screening for herself and her children and referrals to other welfare agencies.

The way that WIC works, is that a woman on the program is given WIC checks or vouchers that she can take to a special WIC store or to her local grocery store. The vouchers specify the items that can be purchased. Once the woman has shopped for the items on the voucher, she would turn in the WIC voucher to the cashier when checking out of the store. WIC foods include infant formula and cereals, cheese, milk, eggs, and adult cereals. Depending on the woman's profile, she may qualify for other WIC items such as peanut butter, beans, carrots and tuna. When you enroll in the program they will tell you what items you may purchase.

To find out about your local WIC program, contact your local health department.

WELFARE-TEMPORARY ASSISTANCE FOR NEEDY FAMILIES

Depending on your financial situation, you may qualify for TANF. TANF is short for Temporary Assistance For Needy Families, which some people simply refer to as welfare benefits. This is the cash aspect of welfare. TANF provides limited assistance to needy families with children to promote work, responsibility and self-sufficiency. TANF provides cash benefits for recipients. The amount of your cash benefits will be determined by the size of your family and other factors, such as if there is other income coming into the home.

If you receive TANF you may automatically qualify for Medicaid and or the Food Stamp program. To apply for TANF, you will need to fill out an application available from your local department of social services. The work component of TANF requires recipients to be working or actively seeking employment. It is meant to be a temporary assistance program. States determine which services/benefits to provide and whom to serve. Cash grants, work opportunities, and other services are provided directly to needy families.

Pregnancy Centers

Pregnancy Centers are facilities that help women who have decided to continue with their pregnancy whether she has decided to place her child up for adoption or if she plans to raise the child on her own. If a woman is considering an abortion, she should not go to a Pregnancy Center because even though they will provide some abortion information, they are far more helpful in helping pregnant women who wish to carry their pregnancy to term than those who plan to abort. These Pregnancy Centers operate under different names such as Crisis Pregnancy Centers, CPC, or other names. They provide women with abortion alternatives. For the woman facing an unplanned pregnancy who has decided to proceed with her pregnancy, a Pregnancy Center can be a wonderful resource and help her in more ways than she could ever imagine.

Pregnancy Centers provide free services to pregnant women. They offer free pregnancy test and a wide range of other services. All services are confidential. The people who work at Pregnancy Centers can offer you a loving shoulder to cry on and can also be strong for you when you feel that you can't carry on. The centers offer counseling services and if a woman needs one, they can have a personal advocate who will work with them throughout their pregnancy.

Education is a big part of the role of the Pregnancy Center. The centers often have guest speakers and they have a collection of books and videos about pregnancy and fetal development.

The Centers also provide referrals for housing, adoption, medical assistance, maternity and infant clothing and equipment. Some Pregnancy Centers even hold baby showers for the women who attend classes at the centers. Classes offered at some of the centers include nutrition, infant CPR, parenting skills, and breast feeding.

To find a nationwide listing of Pregnancy Centers visit-
http://www.pregnancycenters.org/

MATERNITY SHELTERS
You never know if you will find yourself in a situation where housing may become an issue. If you find yourself in need of shelter, there are places that can help you. Pregnant teens may find themselves with no place to go and need to utilize the resources of a maternity shelter. A young woman in an abusive relationship who doesn't have the financial means to get away, but wants to

leave the relationship for the safety of herself and her unborn child may utilize the services of a maternity shelter. A college student who wants to continue her education, but her university doesn't offer family housing may turn to the services of a maternity shelter. The situation may vary, but the services of these shelters are invaluable.

There are maternity shelters for teens and adult women in all 50 states. The services offered and the age range of clients accepted varies from shelter to shelter.

If you are in need of a maternity shelter, they are there and it is best to call several shelters to find one that is best for you. Whereas some shelters only service teens, other service woman of all ages. Many of the shelters have rules that you may find unacceptable, such as curfews or no overnight passes, so it is best that you find a shelter that would work best for your situation. Some shelters also limit the number of children that a client may have, and have restrictions on age limits. Most shelters have limited bed space, so you may have to call around. There also may be a waiting list.

When the word "shelter" is mentioned some people have an automatic image in their head of a low quality place for people in the most desperate of situations. The maternity shelters are often as posh as hotels in some situations. The shelters strive to provide the best living conditions for you and your child. They aim to create an atmosphere that is like a home away from home, although transitional in nature.

The goal of most maternity shelters is to prepare you and your child to be able to live on your own in an apartment or home setting.

Some of the services you may encounter while living in a maternity shelter may include:

- Safe short term housing
- Educational assistance
- Parenting classes
- Substance abuse counseling

- Daycare assistance
- Job training and placement assistance
- Clothing for the mother and the children
- Outreach services
- Independent living skills

Lifecall is a web site dedicated to educating teens and helping pregnant women. They have an on-line directory of maternity shelters, organized state by state.

Additional information
Lifecall Maternity Shelter Listing
http://www.lifecall.org/shelters.html

Public Housing
Public housing is a broad term which can include housing projects, Section 8 housing (now known as the Housing Choice Voucher Program) and much more. Public housing provides decent and safe rental housing to low-income families who meet the eligibility requirements. To qualify for public housing you must meet income requirements, qualify as a family and be an U.S. citizen.

Public housing has a wide array of housing types that include high rises, single family homes, apartments, townhouses and other types of attached housing.

Qualifying for public housing is a somewhat rigorous process but the outcome is well worth it if you are truly in need of low income housing. You will have to submit documentation (birth certificates, tax documents, additional documentation) and participate in interviews and a check of references. The process is in many ways similar to renting an apartment in the private sector. The housing agency will review the information provided. You will be notified whether you are accepted into the public housing program.

You will be expected to pay a security deposit in some situations and you will be informed of what your monthly rent amount will be.

Once you are accepted into the public housing program, technically you can stay in the program as long as you want. However, you must not break any of the rules in your agreement with the housing association and you must continue to meet the income and family requirements of your agreement.

To apply for public housing contact you're local housing agency. The public housing program receives federal aid from The U.S. Department of Housing and Urban Development.

Section 8/Housing Choice Vouchers

Although commonly referred to as Section 8, the Section 8 housing program now falls under a program called Housing Choice Vouchers. This is a program that is a part of the Public Housing Program. The Housing Choice Voucher Program allows low income families to choose where they want to live, versus living in a set housing project unit. With Housing Choice Vouchers low-income families can lease or purchase housing in a neighborhood that is safe and of a decent quality. Housing Choice Vouchers can be used to rent privately owned rental property. The recipient can choose their own housing—which is an advantage to not having an alternative to living in an area that is saturated with low income housing.

To apply for a Housing Choice Voucher you have to apply at your local public housing agency. There are usually waiting lists. When you come to the top of the list you will then receive a voucher. You then can choose your own housing and the public housing agency creates a contract with the landlord or property owner. They pay the landlord or property owner a set portion of the rent and you pay the difference.

PUBLIC HOUSING STORIES

Ona, age 21
"The waiting list for Section 8 where I lived wasn't too bad. Once we were approved and our name came up on the list, I knew just where I wanted to live. I picked a nice townhouse in a really lush family friendly neighborhood. The school districts are good and I can afford my rent. I'm working and taking classes at the community college. My parents didn't have the room at home for me and a baby so Section 8 worked great for me."

Isis age 23
"People always say bad things about living in the projects but my home is nice. The neighbors are a different story. If it weren't for all the people hanging around outside it would be better. I live in a public housing community in Chicago. I can still get around the city because of the busses. I attend classes at a local community college and I plan to be a nurse one day. Whoever manages these projects is really putting a lot of energy into making this a nice place to live."

Maternity Leave
Maternity leave is the name given to the time off a woman takes from work after giving birth. It usually ranges from 4-6 weeks. However, if you make special arrangements with your employer, or have complications with your pregnancy, you can arrange to take a longer or shorter maternity leave.

The bad thing about maternity leave is that most teens and college students don't have jobs that offer maternity leave. Many teens and college students work part time jobs or jobs that don't offer the same type of benefits that many full time positions offer. If you work a part time job, at best your employer may generously hold your job for you or maybe offer you some kind of extended pay program, but the majority of part time jobs do not offer maternity leave benefits to employees.

If you do work full time, your employer most likely will offer you up to six weeks for maternity leave to take care of your newborn child. Don't make the mistake and assume that you automatically get maternity leave. Small companies and certain other types of employers do not have to comply with maternity leave laws. If the company that you work for employs more than 15 people, you cannot be fired if you go on maternity leave. You are protected under the same laws that protect disabled employees. Talk to your employer. This is the best way to find out the options available to you.

Some jobs offer employees a paid 6 week maternity leave. Others may offer employees 50% of their current pay while they are on maternity leave. Some jobs don't offer any kind of financial support towards maternity leave and require that employees use their sick time or vacation time. If you do not have enough sick or vacation time you may have to return to work or continue to take time off in a leave without pay status. Communication is the key. Contact your supervisor or human resources department at least several months prior to your delivery.

Some women can't afford to take the time off for maternity leave, but they will need to in order to bond with their new child and to allow their body time to heal. In rare cases, women will return to work immediately after giving birth.

Most jobs don't want you at work immediately after giving birth. Some jobs require a doctors release before allowing you to return to work.

If your job does not offer a paid maternity leave, and you don't have enough vacation or sick leave to cover your maternity leave, try to discuss other options with your employer. Your company may have a leave sharing program that will allow other employees to donate some of their vacation time to you. Your employer may also allow you to telecommute or work from home during your maternity leave to allow you to keep generating income during your time off.

College work study jobs are often more lenient and compassionate when it comes to letting a student have their old job back after a non required maternity leave. Often work study jobs will give you the time off-unpaid, and allow you to return to work after the requested time off. This is a case by case basis. Some employers also offer an unpaid time off to their part time employees and allow them to come back to work at their same pay grade after their maternity leave.

MATERNITY LEAVE STORIES

Simone, age 19
"I was working as a waitress when I had my daughter. I went into labor on Thursday morning, was released from the hospital Friday, and was back at work Saturday night. People kept trying to scare me and tell me that I would hemorrhage or bleed too much from standing on my feet all day and that my body had to heal. They didn't understand my situation. I was a single parent living in a pay by the week hotel and I had to pay for diapers. My co-workers babysat for free while I worked. "

Gaeda, age 20
"My work study boss was mad cool. They through me a big baby shower two weeks before my due date and they gave me a stroller and a crib. They didn't have a maternity leave program in place for part time workers. They passed an envelope around the office and collected money for me. I was presented me with $400 at the shower. My job was waiting for me when I was ready to come back to work. I only took 4 weeks off because I was going stir crazy sitting around the house with the baby all day. My boyfriend had morning classes so he watched the baby for me while I worked early evening."

Holly, age 21
"I was working as a secretary for a law firm that had three attorneys by day and taking college paralegal courses by night. By law my job didn't have to comply with any maternity leave laws, but they tried to accommodate me. They hired a temp who was

completely lost and called me at home every day. During my time out, they went through 4 temps, who all became overwhelmed and quit. I was running out of money because I only had two weeks of vacation time saved up. I returned to work 3 ½ weeks after having my baby. I needed the job. They said they weren't going to fire me, but they called me at home so much and sounded so frustrated I felt like my job was on the line."

The Family And Medical Leave Act

The Family and Medical Leave Act, passed in 1993, requires employers to provide up to 12 weeks of unpaid leave in cases of personal illness, illnesses of parents, spouses or children and childbirth. This law does not apply to every one or every situation. Companies that employee 50 employees or less do not have to comply. In addition, the person wishing to utilize the benefits of the Family and Medical Leave Act has to have been on the job at least 1 year. Similar to traditional maternity leave, The Family and Medical Leave Act often is not something that teens and college students are eligible for.

The Family Medical Leave Act will protect your job for up to 12 weeks and it will insure that your health benefits will not be canceled—although you may have to pay insurance premiums.

This law is complex and it is important that you understand the procedures for applying for this leave and all of the ends and outs. Talk to your employer or human resources department if you are interested in pursuing the Family and Medical Leave Act.

CHILDCARE
If you work or go to school, you will need someone to care for your child when you are away. Child care can be expensive and a burden, but it is a necessary component of being a parent. There will be times that you have to leave the baby with someone. It is important to plan your child care in advance. Daycare centers often have long waiting lists for infants, therefore it is best to start calling around before your ninth month. If you plan on having a relative or friend care for you baby, make arrangements to sit down

and talk to them beforehand. Determine how you will compensate them for their time.

If you do decide to pay a friend or family member to care for your child, purchase a receipt book and keep accurate records of the amount of money you pay them for child care. You will need their social security number in order to file your taxes properly and to receive a child care credit.

Daycare Centers

Day care centers provide child care to small children. Day care providers will nurture your child, and as your child grows he or she will have an opportunity to interact with other children. Traditional day care centers usually operate between 6AM and 7PM. If you work or go to school in the evenings or on weekends, a traditional day care may not be the ideal child care option for you. Some large cities or cities that have a large military population have day care centers that operate 24 hours a day. Daycare centers are rather expensive. Infant care prices can range from $100-$350 a week depending on the area you live in and the type of daycare center you choose for your child.

Most day care centers begin taking infants at six weeks of age. The majority of day care centers require parents to provide diapers, formula or expressed breast milk and wipes for their infants.

When choosing a day care center make sure that the facility is licensed and that they require background checks on all of their employees. Investigate any prospective day care center. Ask friends and neighbors if they have heard anything about the facility or if they had positive or negative experiences with the facility.

Don't rush to judgement when choosing a day care. Don't choose a facility based on how large their ad is in the phone book or because they always have commercials on television. Arrange to visit the day care prior to enrolling your child. Take a mental note of how the staff interacts with the infants. Also monitor safety conditions at the day care center. Does the front door have a buzzer or secure entry system? Are walkways clear? Do they have a security system and cameras that monitor the classrooms?

Prior to enrolling your child, the day care center may ask you for a deposit to hold your spot. Often times these deposits are non-refundable, so be sure of your decision before paying any type of deposit.

Before choosing to put your child in a traditional day care center, assess your situation. Will the operating hours of the day care center fit within your schedule? If your child becomes sick will you be able to find alternative child care? These are just a few of the questions you should ask yourself when trying to determine what type of child care situation is best for you.

If you receive welfare benefits you may be eligible for subsidized day care benefits. This is something that you should talk to your caseworker about if you are interested.

Home Day Care

Licensed home based day care centers operate similar to traditional day care centers. They have to abide by certain rules regarding the number of children they can care for and their home is subject to inspection by the state. Home day care providers are required to follow strict standards regarding safety, training, nutrition, and the equipment in their homes.

One of the benefits of home day care centers is that they often offer more flexibility than traditional day care centers. One of the downfalls to some home day cares is that when the primary provider is unable to watch the children, you may have to find alternative childcare. Depending on the provider, they may offer evening and weekend child care. Sometimes home day care is less expensive that traditional day care.

Use the same skills that you would use when choosing a traditional day care center when you are looking for a home day care provider. You will need to ask a few more questions of home day care providers. Find out if there will be older children or other adults in the house in the same area where the children will be cared from. Ensure that the provider has safe cribs for infants. If the provider doesn't have cribs or playpens for your child, you may have to provide these. Make sure that the area where the children are being cared for is safe. It is also very important to make sure that the home daycare has insurance.

DAYCARE STORIES

Mira, age 18
"I love my son's babysitter. She interacts with him so well and nurtures him. I am so lucky to have found such a great sitter. What sucks is that when she got mono for two weeks I had to find another sitter for my son. I couldn't find another sitter on such short notice and ended up getting an incomplete in several of my classes because I missed so many days."

Quintasha, age 20
"My daughter's first daycare was a mess. They didn't hold the babies, they didn't change them until they thought the parents were on the way and they called me at least once a week claiming that she was sick—when she wasn't. There was no security, you could walk right in the front door and into the classrooms. I hated that daycare. I didn't realize when I signed the contract that they required a 4 week notice before I could take her out of there. I paid them for a second month and then switched my daughter to a better daycare. The new daycare is $30 a week more expensive but it is worth it because it is so much better."

FEEDING YOUR BABY

Breastfeeding
Breastfeeding is the easiest way to feed your new baby. It's cheaper than bottle feeding and it's convenient. The American Academy of Pediatrics determined that breast milk is the ideal nutrition for your babies first twelve months of life.

Some women are apprehensive about breast feeding due to things they have heard from families and friends. If you deliver your baby in a hospital, many hospitals have lactation consultants that can assist you with breastfeeding. If the hospital you deliver at has no lactation consultant available, a nurse may be able to help you with breastfeeding basics such as helping your baby latch on to your breast.

Breastfeeding has little to do with the size of your breasts, so don't think that the size of your breasts will determine if you will be able to breast feed or not. If you carried your baby to term and your breasts produced milk, you should be able to breast feed.

Even if you are going to be a working mom or a mom that goes to school, you can still choose to nurse your baby. Your breast milk can be expressed into a bottle by hand or with a breast pump.

The La Leche League International is an organization dedicated to providing information and support to women who choose to breast feed. You can look in your phone book or visit the La Leche Leagues web site to find a Le Leche League group in your area. If there is no La Leche League in your area, your doctor, local health department or a Pregnancy Center may be able to assist your with breastfeeding basics.

Formula Feeding

Don't feel like a failure if breastfeeding is not for you. Millions of women formula feed their babies every year and they thrive and grow into healthy toddlers. Formula feeding can cost you up to $1200 a year. If you are on the WIC program, they will be able to provide you with infant formula for free. When choosing a formula, select an iron fortified formula. There are many different brands on the market, but they are similar. Choose one formula for your infant and only switch formula if your doctor suggests that your infant change formula.

Many of the popular infant formulas give out coupons and free samples. By visiting their web sites you can often sign up for their mailing lists.

The directions are right on the container. There are several types of formula that you can choose from:

- Powder-The powder formula has to be mixed with water. Directions are included on the canister. The powder is usually the least expensive method to use over a long period of time.

- Concentrate-The concentrate infant formula has to be mixed with water. Directions are included on the bottle.

- Ready To Feed-The ready to feed infant formula is the easiest to use. The formula is ready to use and does not have to be mixed. Although, the most convenient, this type of formula can be the most expensive choice if used over a long period of time.

AFTER THE BABY

After your baby is born, you may find yourself overwhelmed. Now you will be the mother of a new little person who will depend on you for their every need. Whether this is your first child or a second or third, every new child will require your love and attention. The birth of a new child can be a joyous and a stressful time.

If you find yourself feeling very sad and depressed after the birth of your child you may be developing postpartum depression. Postpartum depression refers to the mental state of a woman following the birth of a child. If you feel hopeless or sad it is important that you contact your health care provider. This is a treatable condition.

STORIES OF UNPLANNED PREGNANCIES

Marisa, age 19   My High School Sweetheart

"Justin was my high school sweetheart. He was a year ahead of me, so when I was a junior he was a senior looking forward to graduation and college. He had a football scholarship and was going to college several states away. We planned to stay close through e-mail and holiday breaks. I never thought Justin and I would break up.

Justin left for college in August. Soon after he left, I discovered that I was pregnant. As soon as he arrived at college, I didn't really hear from him anymore. He told me he was busy with school and football so I believed him. When I told him I was pregnant, he told me that I was lying and that it probably wasn't his because he had been gone almost a month.

I became so sad and depressed. I did consider having an abortion, but I didn't have any money and I was too embarrassed to tell me dad that I was pregnant. I managed to scrape up enough money to catch the Greyhound bus to Ohio to visit Justin—a trip that took over a day and was hundreds of miles from my home in Minnesota. When I arrived at his dorm, he hung up the phone when I told him I was outside of his building.

I sat outside of the dorm crying when I met some girls that went to Justin's school. If it wasn't for them I don't know what I would have done. They let me stay with them. Justin did finally agree to see me, but when we met in his dorm room, it was not good. The girls I met gave me money for a bus ticket and I went back home. I managed to tell my father that I was pregnant and he was supportive. I gave birth to a precious baby girl. Justin has only seen the baby through pictures. He is still in college, so I don't get any child support from him. I don't regret having my little girl. I do wish that Justin and I could be together as a couple."

Keisha, age 16   **Someone Else To Think About**

"My story is straight stupid. My babies daddy is just a jerk. We hooked up when I was 15 and he was 17. He told me that his ex-girlfriend had aborted his baby and that is why they broke up. He told me that he would love to have a baby by me because I was pretty and light-skinned and that our baby would look so pretty. Why was I so dumb? I wasn't trying to get pregnant, but let's put it like this—I wasn't doing much to prevent it. We never used protection and when I became pregnant he was happy.

When the baby came everything changed. He still wanted to hang out with his friends. He would drop off diapers and small amounts of money, but he never helped me take care of the baby. We would argue all the time and we broke up. He now has a new girlfriend-who is pregnant. He works at the grocery store and I get child support—$123 a month, which is not much at all, but I guess it's better than nothing. I love my daughter, and he loves her also. I definitely wish I would have waited. It is very, very hard to be a high school student and a mother. My family helps me, but I feel like I am missing out on a lot of things. Most of my friends have babies, but I always have to think about my daughter. I can't just think about Keisha anymore. It's tough."

Debbie, age 19   **It's Working**

"Have you ever heard the story about the girl who lost her virginity on her prom night and got pregnant? Yeah, I bet you missed that one. That's what happened to me. My boyfriend and I had been together for four years and I promised him that we would go "all the way" on prom night.

Our inexperience was a problem because the condom broke and he didn't even realize it. I didn't know about the morning after pill, and I became pregnant. I was planning on going away to college and my boyfriend was planning on going to the Air Force.

We changed our plans around big time. He still enlisted in the Air Force, but we got married much sooner than we had planned. We had always said that if our relationship survived 4 years of college that we would tie the knot. The military has good benefits and we live in military family housing. I enrolled in several college courses and our daughter goes to day care.

I feel like such a grown up now. I cook dinner, change diapers, and iron my husbands uniform. I feel sad sometimes when I talk to my friends from home and they are telling me about college parties and sororities and all the things I am missing out on, but I made this decision for myself and I have to live with it. Sometimes I wonder what would have happened if I would have had an abortion, but I love my family and I am glad that I chose this path for myself."

Roshumba, age 17   It's Not All Bad

"I felt compelled to share my story because it's not all bad when teens get pregnant. I became pregnant at age 14. It was very hard and difficult being a mother at such a young age. My boyfriend and I stayed together, we never broke up—although we did have some heated arguments. I now volunteer and speak to other teens about teen pregnancy prevention. I graduate next year and am going to college. The university I was accepted to has family housing and my boyfriend has an athletic scholarship to the same school so we will continue to raise our child together."

Nadia, age-22   Consequences

"Grady and I had a strictly sexual relationship. We were both juniors in college. I knew he had a girlfriend out there in the world somewhere, but when he and I were together, our time together was really special. I was in love and I didn't take my pills on schedule because I felt like if I got pregnant by Grady everything would be alright.

Well everything wasn't alright. It was winter time when I found out that I was pregnant. I told Grady and he snapped. He was angry, he said I was trying to mess up the good thing that we had, and that it probably wasn't his. He immediately cut off our relationship. He wouldn't take my calls and whenever I went to his dorm room his roommate said he wasn't there.

My due date was in August. Grady went home for summer break in May and I was hoping that over the summer he would have an opportunity to think about things and he would come around. When school started, Grady was no where to be found. Much to my surprise, he transferred to a school 1000 miles away. Who would transfer during their senior year?

I finished college and started a teaching job the following year. Grady agreed to a paternity test after he was served him with child support papers and I now get child support. I love my daughter. He has never seen her, but he is the one missing out."

CHAPTER 3-BABY GEAR—WHAT TO BUY NOW AND WHAT CAN WAIT

NEW BABY ITEM CHECKLIST
It's inevitable. You have a new baby on the way and you have to prepare. Friends, family members, even magazines and books will influence your purchases. People will tell you what you need and what you absolutely can't do without. Baby equipment and gear is expensive, so you will want to plan your purchases well.

<u>MUST HAVE</u>
You may have a pre-set notion of your must have items, but here is a handy guide with suggested purchases that will get you started.

Car Seat
You need a car seat to get your baby home from the hospital so a car seat should be one of the first items that you invest in. Although many items you can purchase second hand, it is usually best to invest in a new car seat. There are several styles available. Some styles convert into infant carriers that make transporting the baby inside the vehicle and around town convenient. There are also larger car seats that can be used until the child is a toddler. The larger car seats also can be used as rear facing car seats. The infant carrier car seats are convenient but usually by the time the baby is 9-12 months old it time for a new car seat. If you do purchase an infant carrier car seat, be prepared to buy a larger car seat in the future.

Crib
You need a crib. Older family members may tell you stories about how you or other babies in the family did fine sleeping in the bed with them, but safety is paramount. Although rare, there have been situations where parents rolled onto small babies causing them to smother. Adult size beds are not made for babies, it is easy for babies to smother in soft bedding or to get caught between the

headboard and the mattress. Purchasing a crib is your best bet. When choosing a crib, make sure that the crib is of a high quality and that all of the pieces are affixed properly. If you purchase a crib second hand make sure that all pieces are included and that the crib meets current safety standards.

Clothes

You are going to need clothes for your baby. If you have a baby shower, request that family and friends purchase clothes of various sizes. Newborn size clothing won't last long. Babies grow very fast. If you have some newborn size clothing along with 3-6 months and 6-9 months clothing you should be fine for the first few months. Spend your money wisely. Buy clothing that will be season appropriate. If your baby is due in the summer, don't stock up on winter clothes. Who knows what size your baby will be wearing by that time? Shop wisely. High end department stores often have just one baby outfit priced at $25. Discount chains such as Walmart or Target often offer baby clothes priced much lower. Also check consignment and resell shops. Nothing is wrong with splurging for a nice outfit for baby's homecoming or for a special event, but your dollars will go further if you buy less expensive clothes.

Blankets

Blankets are a must. There will be times when you need to wrap the baby up inside of the house or when you are out and about. Babies also like to feel snug and secure and will appreciate being swaddled or wrapped tight in a blanket. You don't have to spend a lot of money on receiving blankets. Often you can purchase a pack of three receiving blankets for under $10. If you know someone who crochets or knits they may be able to make you a few blankets if you purchase the supplies for them.

Diapers

Whether you use disposable diapers or order a diaper service and use cloth diapers, diapers are a must have. If you purchase diapers prior to your child's birth, don't stock up on too many newborn or small size diapers. Babies grow very fast!

Wipes

Wipes make cleaning up messy diapers a snap. Although a warm towel does the job, wipes are convenient, especially if you have to change the baby while you are out and about.

Bottles

Whether you breastfeed or bottle feed bottles are a must. If you breastfeed, you may need to pump breast milk into a bottle so that whoever takes care of the baby in your absence can feed the baby. You can't bottle feed without bottles. Don't be tricked into buying the most expensive brand. Bottles found at the dollar store are often just as good as name brand bottles. Sometimes you can find the name brand bottles at the dollar store. However, if you invest in one good set of bottles they may last longer.

Baby Bathtub

Baby bath tubs make giving baby a bath easy. Many will tell you that washing the baby in the sink is just as efficient, but a baby bath will offer you the support to prop up the baby as you clean the infant. Many of the baby baths on the market convert into toddler tubs. Baby baths can be purchased for usually under twenty dollars. You shouldn't leave the baby alone in the baby bath, but baby baths still offer more support than a sink or bucket.

CAN WAIT

It may seem exciting to stock up on baby gear, but you aren't going to need everything right away. Some baby equipment you won't need until the baby is a little bit older so it's okay to budget your purchases.

Stroller

If you purchased a car seat that converts into an infant carrier you might be able to hold off a few months on buying a stroller. The infant carrier is ideal for taking the baby to the doctor, the grocery store or on short trips. If you do a lot of walking it would probably be a good ideal to purchase a stroller sooner than later. As with car seats, strollers vary in price. An umbrella stroller can often be purchased for less than $15 but the strollers that recline and have various amenities have a price range of $45 to $300 or more.

Digital Camera or Video Camera
Naturally baby is here and you want to catch every exciting moment on film. If you can't afford an expensive camera don't fret. Until you have the money, purchase disposable cameras. A disposable camera can be purchased for less than $10 and most produce high quality pictures. You can still email pictures to family and friends if when you have them developed you ask them to put the pictures on a CD-ROM or some developers have the on-line pictures option. The on-line picture option allows you to have hard copies of your pictures and a link to where your pictures can be found on-line.

Play Pen or Pack And Play
If you have a crib, you probably won't have much use for your pack and play in the beginning. For this reason, this is something that can wait until baby is a little older. If you need to contain the baby while you are in another room, an infant carrier should be okay or if you have plush carpet you can put down a blanket and let baby entertain himself on the floor.

High Chair
Your baby won't be ready to sit in the high chair until he or she can sit up on their own. So you probably won't have much need for a high chair until your baby is at least 4-6 months old.

Toys
It's nice to have a mobile over the crib or other infant toys for stimulation and enjoyment but when the baby first comes home he

or she isn't going to be playing with many toys. Blocks, cars, dolls, and educational toys can wait until baby is a little older.

Baby food and eating utensils
Your baby won't be eating solid foods when he or she first comes home from the hospital, so you can hold off on stocking up on baby food.

OPTIONAL
Some mothers will tell you they couldn't imagine having raised their child without these items, but trust, your baby will be just fine if you don't have these items.

Bassinet
Bassinets are beautiful and some mothers like the idea of having the bassinet in the same room with them verses a big crib. If you can afford one (and if your baby will sleep in it), bassinets are an okay investment. The bad thing about a bassinet is that they are only safe until a baby can turn over. So once your baby is over the specified weight for safe use of the bassinets or can turn over, the bassinet has to be retired. For this reason, a crib is a much better investment, you will get much more use out of it.

Changing Table
A changing table is a nice piece of furniture if you can afford it but you can change your baby sufficiently on the bed or the floor. Additionally, the changing table often becomes just something that you sit items on when your baby becomes too mobile to change on the changing tables.

Infant Swings and Rocking Chairs
Baby swings and rocking chairs are nice to have and they often help lull baby to sleep but if you can't afford it your baby will be just as content going to sleep in your arms.

Bottle Warmers and Sterilizers

Bottle warmers and sterilizers can be expensive investments although there are cheaper brands on the market. It is not advised that you microwave a babies bottle but there are a number of ways to warm a bottle rather than using a bottle warmer. Bottle warmers are convenient but running a bottle under warm water is just as effective. Boiling water to clean bottles or using a home dishwasher will work as sufficient as a sterilizer.

Humidifiers and Vaporizer

Unless your doctor recommends a humidifier or a vaporizer for health reasons your baby will be just fine breathing the same air as you.

Expensive cremes, lotions and powders

Other mothers or family members may swear by certain brands but expensive lotions, cremes and powders can be costly. If you find a generic brand that works just as good it should work just as good on baby. If you notice your child has an allergic reaction to a certain brand it would be a good idea to switch brands, but the most expensive brand doesn't always mean that it is the best available.

Chapter 4-Continuing Your Education and Parenting

Just because you are having a baby doesn't mean that your education is over. No matter what your education or career goals were before you became a parent you can still achieve those goals—although you might have to work a little harder.

FINISHING HIGH SCHOOL
Now more than ever it is capable for a young woman to be a mother and a student. Some high schools that have a large population of teenage mothers offer in school day care centers. In school day care is a controversial topic among educators. Some believe that by offering child care to young mothers it will encourage teens to go ahead and have a baby, knowing that they can still go to the same school and their social life may not be altered much. Others believe that by offering child care more teen mothers will complete their high school education. A study completed by the Elizabeth Celotto Child Care Center at Wilbur Cross High School found that none of the teen mothers in their program had repeat births while in the program. The mothers utilizing the program also were shown to have better school performance and that the mothers were paid extra special attention to making sure that their children's immunizations records were up to date. The Elizabeth Celotto Child Care Center provides child care for up to 32 infant and toddlers while their mothers attend classes at the high school.

The best way to find out if your school district has a high school that offers in school child care is to call the school board or your school district's main office.

If there is no school in your area that offers in school child care, there are other programs that can help you finish school. As mentioned in a previous chapter, there are subsidized programs that can help you obtain reasonable child care. If you don't qualify for a subsidized program you have the option of finding a babysitter or daycare program to care for your child while you attend classes.

School districts are starting to offer more flexible programs for high school students to finish their high school education. They are realizing that more and more students have extenuating circumstances that might not allow them to go to school in a regular 6 hour school day setting. Some school districts offer night classes and home school programs. If these options sound like something you may be interested in pursuing check with your local school district.

COMPLETING YOUR HIGH SCHOOL DIPLOMA VIA DISTANCE LEARNING

Distance learning is learning that occurs outside of a traditional classroom setting. Distance learning can involve instruction from various methods including correspondence courses, on-line courses, or a combination of traditional or multimedia delivery methods. Distance learning is a good way for you to complete your high school diploma if you are a self-starter and someone who can stay motivated without a teacher always around. Most distance learning programs allow the students flexibility in completing their assignments. Assignments are usually due at a certain time or date but you can work on the assignments during a time that is convenient for you.

As there are college programs that will allow you to complete your degree online, there are also programs that will allow you to complete your high school diploma on-line. If you are interested in finishing your high school diploma on-line there are several things you need to look for in a program. You first of all want to make sure that the program is accredited. Getting your diploma from an accredited program ensures that your diploma will be recognized by future employers, colleges, universities, technical schools and the military.

Accredited On-Line High School Diploma Programs

Christa McAuliffe Academy
2520 W. Washington Ave
Yakima, Washington, 98903
1-866-575-4989
http://www.cmacademy.org

Keystone National High School
420 West 5th St.
Bloomsburg, PA 17815-1564
1-800-255-4937
http://www.keystonehighschool.com

These are just examples of two accredited on-line learning programs that offer high school diplomas. There are many available that you can find by searching the Internet.

If you do not have the type of access to the Internet necessary to complete your high school diploma on-line you can complete your diploma via a correspondence program. Although correspondence programs have faltered some in popularity due to the increase in Internet based high school diploma programs, there are still programs that will allow you to complete your assignments via the U.S. mail system.

American School is one of the nations oldest accredited correspondence schools that will allow you to complete your high school diploma. They will give you credit for any previous high school work as long as your previous program was accredited. They offer two high school programs, their General High School Course and their College Preparatory Course.

American School
2200 East 170th Street
Lansing, IL 60438
www.americanschoolofcorr.com

American School is just one example of a high school correspondence school. There are others available.

Most distance learning high school diploma programs give you a certain amount of time to complete the program. Some also have convenient payment plans.

GED-GENERAL EDUCATIONAL DEVELOPMENT TEST

GED is short for general educational development test. A passing score on the GED test will give you the equivalent of a high school diploma. If you are unable to complete high school in an on campus setting or via distance learning, obtaining a GED might be a good idea. If you successfully pass the GED exam, you will have the same credentials as someone who completes high school in a traditional manner. The GED exam is made up of five tests that will test your knowledge in the following areas: Interpreting literature and the arts, math, social studies, science and writing. You will be able to use your GED to get a job, continue your education at a college, university, or technical school or enter the military.

The route to getting your GED is up to you. There are programs that will allow you to take classes to prepare you for taking the test. If getting to a class is not an option, you can study at home with books, CD-ROM's or various other test preparation methods. However, for the actual test you will have to take it in person at a testing center or location.

Prometrics is a company that offers nationwide GED testing. They are only one avenue to getting your GED. They have testing centers nationwide. There also may be GED programs in your area offered from community colleges and high school.

Prometrics GED Online
www.prometric.com

GOING TO COLLEGE?

It used to be when a young woman had a child she couldn't go away to college. Colleges and universities didn't create environments that fostered parenthood. If a woman did have a child she had to live in an apartment off campus. Now a great deal of colleges and universities offer family housing. Family housing provides housing for single and married students who have children. Some universities allow unmarried couples to live in family housing. The specific requirements to qualify to live in family housing vary by school. Some universities require students in family housing to maintain certain academic standards (usually just passing grades). Others place requirements on age or year in school, (such as allowing students 19 and up to live in family housing or sophomore status and up). At the same time, there are many schools that allow freshman with dependent children to apply to live in family housing. Below is a listing of colleges and universities that offer family housing. For space sake, only one-two schools are listed per state, but just because you don't see your school of interest listed doesn't mean that they don't offer family housing. This list is by no means all inclusive, it's just to get you started!

U.S. COLLEGES AND UNIVERSITIES THAT OFFER FAMILY HOUSING

ALABAMA
University of Alabama at Huntsville
http://housing.uah.edu/

Troy State University
http://www.troyst.edu/housing/reshalls.html

ALASKA
University of Alaska-Fairbanks
http://www.uaf.edu/reslife/family/

University of Alaska Southeast
http://www.uas.alaska.edu/housing/

ARIZONA
Arizona State University East
http://www.east.asu.edu/housing/

Northern Arizona State University
http://www4.nau.edu/reslife/reslife/

ARKANSAS
Arkansas State University
http://reslife.astate.edu/

CALIFORNIA
Berkley
http://www.housing.berkeley.edu/

University of California Davis
http://www.housing.ucdavis.edu/

COLORADO
University of Colorado at Boulder
http://www-housing.colorado.edu/

University of Northern Colorado
http://housing.unco.edu/

CONNECTICUT
University of Connecticut
http://www.reslife.uconn.edu/

DELAWARE
University of Delaware
http://www.udel.edu/has/

FLORIDA
Florida State
http://www.housing.fsu.edu/

University of Florida
http://www.housing.ufl.edu/

GEORGIA
Georgia Tech
http://tenthandhome.housing.gatech.edu/

University of Georgia
http://www.uga.edu/housing

HAWAII
BYU Hawaii
http://w3.byuh.edu/housing/

IDAHO
Idaho State University
http://www.isu.edu/housing/

Boise State University
http://housing.boisestate.edu/

ILLINOIS
Southern Illinois University at Carbondale
http://www.housing.siu.edu/

University of Illinois at Champaign-Urbana
http://www.housing.uiuc.edu/

INDIANA
Indiana State University
http://www.indstate.edu/reslife

IOWA
Iowa State
http://www.iastate.edu/

KANSAS
Kansas State University
http://www.housing.k-state.edu

The University of Kansas
http://www.housing.ku.edu

KENTUCKY
Eastern Kentucky University
http://www.housing.eku.edu

University of Kentucky
http://www.uky.edu/Housing

LOUISIANA
Louisiana State University
http://www.lsu.edu/housing

Nicholls State University
http://www.nicholls.edu/

MAINE
University of Maine
http://sas.umaine.edu/housing/

MARYLAND
No listing

MASSACHUSETTS
Massachusetts Institute of
Technology
http://web.mit.edu/housing/

University of Massachusetts at
Amherst
http://www.housing.umass.edu/family/index.html

MICHIGAN
Michigan State University
http://www.hfs.msu.edu/uh/

Northern Michigan University
http://www.nmu.edu/housing/

MINNESOTA
University of Minnesota
http://www.housing.umn.edu/

MISSISSIPPI
Mississippi State University
http://www.housing.msstate.edu/

University of Southern Mississippi
http://www.usm.edu/pinehaven/

MISSOURI
University of Missouri-Columbia
http://reslife.missouri.edu

MONTANA
Montana State University-Billings
http://www.msubillings.edu/reslife/

Montana Tech The University of
Montana
http://www.mtech.edu/housing/

NEBRASKA
Creighton University
http://www.creighton.edu/ResidenceLife/

NEBRASKA cont.
University of Nebraska-Lincoln
http://www.unl.edu/housing/family.htm

NEVADA
University of Nevada at Reno
http://www.reslife.unr.edu/village.asp

NEW HAMPSHIRE
University of New Hampshire
http://www.unh.edu/housing/

NEW JERSEY
Rutgers-New Brunswick
http://housing.rutgers.edu/

Rutgers-Newark
http://newark.rutgers.edu/~reslife/

NEW MEXICO
University of New Mexico
http://www.unm.edu/~reshalls/studentFamilyHousing.html

NEW YORK
Syracuse University
http://housingmealplans.syr.edu/

NORTH CAROLINA
North Carolina State University
http://www.ncsu.edu/housing/

NORTH DAKOTA
University of North Dakota
http://www.housing.und.edu/

OHIO
Ohio State University
http://www.buckeyevillage.com/

OKLAHOMA
South Western Oklahoma State
University
http://www.swosu.edu/

OREGON
Southern Oregon University
http://www.sou.edu/housing/

PENNSYLVANIA
Penn State University Park
http://www.hfs.psu.edu/housing/

RHODE ISLAND
No listing

SOUTH CAROLINA
University of South Carolina
http://www.housing.sc.edu/

Winthrop University
http://www.winthrop.edu/reslife/

SOUTH DAKOTA
University of South Dakota
http://www.usd.edu/reslife/fsh/

TENNESSEE
University of Tennessee at
Knoxville
http://uthousing.utk.edu/

TEXAS
University of Texas at Austin
http://www.utexas.edu/student/hous
ing

UTAH
Bringham Young University
http://www.byu.edu/familyhousing/

VERMONT
University of Vermont
http://www.uvm.edu/~reslife/

VIRGINIA
University of Virginia
http://www.virginia.edu/housing/

WASHINGTON
University of Washington
http://hfs.washington.edu/

Central Washington University
http://www.cwu.edu/~housing/

WEST VIRGINIA
Marshall University
http://www.marshall.edu/residence-
services/

West Virginia University
http://www.sa.wvu.edu/housing

WISCONSIN
University of Wisconsin-Madison
http://www.housing.wisc.edu/

WYOMING
University of Wyoming
http://uwadmnweb.uwyo.edu/reslif
e-dining/

Chapter 5- Everything You Ever Wanted To Know About DNA Paternity Testing

A paternity test is often referred to as a DNA test. Daytime television talk shows have somewhat trivialized and made a mockery of DNA testing. Having a DNA test performed is a very serious and somewhat costly measure to take. If you find that you are in a situation where a paternity test is considered it can lead to peace of mind or resolution to a very serious matter.

It happens quite often. A guy and a girl are in a committed (or not so committed) relationship. The young woman discovers that she is pregnant and the guy decides he wants a paternity test. Or else the baby is born and the guy or his family says the baby doesn't look like the father.

The young woman may here the following:

"I want a DNA test."

If your boyfriend asks you for a DNA test and you know that he is the only man you have been sexually active with this can be a very painful time in your life. If you have been sexually active with more than one man and are not sure of who the child's father is, it may be your decision to obtain a DNA test.

DNA Testing Q & A

What is a DNA Test?
DNA testing refers to the process of examining an individual's DNA markers for the purpose of genetic human identification and for determining the relationship between two people.

Who needs to be tested?
The mother, the child and the alleged father. The test can be performed without the mother's sample, but this requires additional

47

analysis and may take a few days longer for the results to be obtained.

How accurate are the test results?
The test results are over 99.999% when determining paternity. If the alleged father's DNA and the child's DNA do not match, he is 100% excluded as the father.

How is the test performed?
The test is performed by taking a Buccal Swab of the inside of the cheeks of the mother, child and alleged father. A DNA analysis can also be performed on a blood sample. The Buccal swab method has grown in popularity because it offers results just as accurate and is non invasive. No blood has to be drawn and it's relatively painless, at most just the slight discomfort of having ones cheek interior swabbed. The sample from the swab is then tested in a lab and the results are obtained.

How long does it take to obtain the results.
It all depends on the lab and the method of testing. Some labs promise results in two weeks or less and others for an express fee can have results in 3 days or less.

How much does the test cost?
Most standard legally binding lab DNA tests start at $400 and up. The standard DNA test usually involves the testing of the child, the mother and the alleged father. If the test requires special analysis such as the testing of only the alleged father and the child, those tests require more in depth analysis and may cost slightly more.

If I leave the baby with the alleged father for a short amount of time can he get the child tested without my permission?
Some lab tests require that the mother sign a release giving permission for the child to be tested or require the alleged father to produce documentation that he has custody or is the custodial parent.

Not all lab tests require the mother to participate or give permission for the test to be performed. Home DNA tests do not require the mother's permission so it is quite possible that the alleged father can arrange a DNA test without the mothers knowledge.

If a home DNA test is performed without my knowledge are the results admissible in a court of law?
No. Lab DNA testing, also known as a legal DNA test, has several steps involved which can include finger printing, photocopying of identification, signed affidavits, and strict monitoring of all samples. This strict monitoring of the testing process is known as chain of custody. A home DNA test does not include this rigorous process, so the results are not admissible in a court of law for most home DNA tests. It is the chain of custody of the samples and properly identifying the parties that makes the home DNA test non admissible.

Why does the mother have to be tested?
In DNA testing, the testers look for several things. The child will share one band with the mother and one band with the father. If the child shares no band with the alleged father, he is excluded as the father. The legal lab DNA test can be performed without the mother also, it is just usually slightly more expensive.

Do I have to wait for the baby to be a certain age before I can get a DNA test?
No. You can have a DNA test performed as soon as the baby is involved. There is even umbilical cord testing available from some DNA labs.

Are home DNA test accurate?
Most home DNA companies claim that their tests are as accurate as lab tests. However, their results are not admissible in court. If

you are going to spend the money for a DNA test it would probably be in your best interest to seek out a legal lab test.

Can we get a test before the baby is born?
Yes. If possible it is better to wait until after the baby is born to have a DNA analysis. The test can be performed prior to the child's birth with Chorionic Villi Sample (CVS), or amniocentesis. Both of these procedures are invasive and can possibly cause risk to the pregnancy. These procedures have to be performed by an OB/GYN. The sample collected can then be submitted for DNA analysis. If you have a high risk pregnancy you may not be a candidate for prenatal DNA testing. If you are interested in prenatal DNA testing it is best that you discuss this with your doctor.

Will the DNA results hold up in court?
DNA test results are usually more that 99.99% accurate in establishing paternity and 100% accurate when excluding paternity. If your test was legally performed by an accredited lab the results will hold up in court. As mentioned previously, home DNA test results are not admissible in court.

Does public aid pay for paternity test?
Every state has different laws on paternity testing associated with their public aid department or program. In some states, if the mother is receiving public assistance, she must participate in determining the paternity of the father if the paternity is in question. This is because some states public aid departments enforce child support. If the mother is getting public aid benefits such as medical assistance, Food Stamps and cash assistance, the state will go after the father for child support. The mother may not see this child support in her hand every month—she may see some of the money or none at all. The state will collect the child support to off set costs for providing services for the mother and child. The state will take various methods to determine paternity.

If there is a doubt about who the father is or if the alleged father has doubt the state can order genetic testing to determine paternity. Sometimes the cost of the test is based on the fathers income. If he can afford the test he may be ordered to pay all or a portion of the cost for the test. If he can't afford the test, he may have to pay a reduced amount or nothing at all. If the alleged father refuses to participate after being served with papers, in some cases, paternity can be established by default. It is best to check with your state public aid office.

The role public aid plays in determining paternity varies state by state.

Will my insurance pay for a DNA test?
Most insurance companies do not pay for DNA testing to determine paternity. However, every insurance company is different. Your best bet would be to check with your insurance company.

How do I choose a DNA test company?
You want to make sure that the company is registered by the AABB, which is short for the American Association of Blood Banks. Although not a necessity, it wouldn't hurt to choose a lab that runs their tests twice. You also want a center that will provide you with an affidavit, expert testimony or depositions if you should need to use your test results for legal reasons. Below are several well respected DNA testing companies.

American Medical Services Corporation
Phone: 866-Are-U-Dad (273-8323)
Fax: 908-820-8932
E-mail: ams@paternitytesters.com
http://www.paternitytesters.com/

DNA Diagnostics Center
205 Corporate Court
Fairfield, OH 45014 USA
Toll Free: (800) 613-5768
E-mail: dna@dnacenter.com
Internet: www.dnacenter.com

Genelex Corporation
3000 First Ave., Suite One
Seattle, WA 98121
Phone-800-523-3080
http://www.genelex.com/

Stories of Paternity Testing

Giselle, age 17

"I am seventeen years old and I am a mother to a handsome little boy named Ivan. I started dating Ivan's father Xavier when I was a sophomore in high school. Our relationship started out casual, just kicking it around the neighborhood. He got kicked out of school for fighting or something stupid and that is when our relationship became sexual. I started cutting school several days a month and would spend days over at his house while his parents worked. I had only had one sexual partner before him and did worry about getting pregnant but he assured me he would "pull out." He didn't believe in condoms.

We talked about having a baby and getting married one day so the few times he didn't pull out I didn't worry because deep inside I felt like everything was going to be okay. My period didn't come three months in a row. I told him I thought I was pregnant. We went to the clinic and found out I was pregnant.

We were happy, it was like our little secret but when his family found out things changed. He stopped taking my calls and became distant. Then he told me his brother said I sleep around and the baby might not be his.

We got over our little spats and he was with me every day towards the end of the pregnancy but when the baby was born he had the nerve to say it wasn't his because his family said it didn't look like him and he wanted a paternity test.

Xavier wanted the test but he didn't offer to pay for it. I called around for a paternity test and the price was $500 where we live. Xavier wasn't a total jerk he brought by diapers from time to time but by this time he was dating someone else. To make a long story short, I ended up getting on welfare when Ivan was 5 months old. The financial burden was too much on my parents. I gave Xavier's name to the welfare people and they arranged for a paternity test. A court ordered DNA test proved Xavier was the father.

He apologized afterwards and said he wanted us to be a family. He broke up with the girl he was dating. I try because I want us to be a family, but it just hurts so bad that he needed a DNA test to accept his own child."

Tiffany, age 22

"College was the best time of my life. I suppose I should say is because I am still in school, it's just I am not having the carefree time I one was. I got caught up in a little bit of drama. I blame a lot of my problems on being young and away from home for the first time—and indulging in a bit too much alcohol.

I was dating a frat boy named Red. He was my creep creep. Our relationship was all sex. He would stop by my dorm after parties, we would get our freak on and that was it. We would smile as we crossed paths on campus and I was cool with that. No shame in my game.

I met a nice boy, a real well bred football player named Drake. Didn't drink, didn't smoke, but he was cute. I met him after a football game around homecoming. We hung out, he had money, he always fed me. Drake and I really started to get close and intimate. I didn't stop seeing Red in the beginning, we were still messing around.

Then things got a bit sticky. Next thing you know, I find out Drake heard through the grapevine that Red and I had been messing around. I tell him that we were, but it is now over. Drake forgave me as long as I promised to leave Red alone for good.

I missed my November period. Between the time of homecoming in October and Thanksgiving I had had sex with Drake and Fred. I wasn't going to say anything. I was just going to say it was Drake's because I knew he would be a better father than Red. Plus I had been having sex with Red all that time and never got pregnant. It would have to be Drake. I was on the pill but would forget to take it 4 or 5 days in a row.

I waited until Valentines Day to tell Drake I was pregnant. He was happy, we talked about getting engaged, then when we went to the doctor together (a mistake on my part) and they told him I was like13-14 weeks, the wheels started turning in his head that it might be Red's.

I promised him the baby was his, and he promised he would be with me no matter what. Red had a girlfriend that he had been with for years, so I knew he wasn't trying to be my baby daddy.

The baby was born, a little girl I named Draya, I thought Drake would forget about the paternity test but he didn't, paid for that joint with his American Express card. It was simple, they swabbed our cheeks and Draya's cheeks. He even sprung for the extra $150 three business day turnaround time.

Those three days were horrible, the waiting, the not knowing. When the test results came back, it turned out that Drake wasn't the father. No more wedding plans, no more engagement, no more I'll be there no matter what. Guys lie. I had to fight with Red to get him to take a paternity test. He finally got tested and the test proved that he was the father. He pays child support, but not much—$60 a month is all the judge ordered because he is a full time student on financial aid working a 10 hour a week work study job. The judge didn't order him to get a full time job because he said that he would have greater future earning power with his degree."

CHAPTER 6- ABORTION-ANSWERS TO YOUR QUESTIONS

Not every young woman who finds herself facing an unplanned pregnancy is going to follow through with the pregnancy and have a child. Abortion is a legal procedure in the country, although having access to a clinic that performs abortions can be a challenge depending on what part of the country you live in. Hopefully, this chapter will clear up any questions or misconceptions that you may have about the abortion procedure.

<u>WHAT IS ABORTION?</u>

Abortion is defined as the termination of a pregnancy. 50% of all unplanned pregnancies result in an abortion. The term induced abortion is used to describe any procedure that results in termination and expulsion of a fetus. Abortion became legal in the United States in January of 1973 when the United States Supreme Court handed down the Roe V. Wade decision allowing women to seek legal abortions. Abortion is a common procedure and many women choose abortion to end an unplanned pregnancy. Despite all of the conflict surrounding this controversial procedure, abortion is still legal in the United States.

Any woman wishing to terminate her pregnancy before 24 weeks of gestation may seek an abortion in the United States. Pregnancy occurs in three stages. The first stage is known as the first trimester. The first trimester is considered between 1-12 weeks of pregnancy. The second stage of pregnancy is known as the second trimester. The second trimester ranges from 12-24 weeks of pregnancy. Abortion is a legal procedure up until the 24 week mark and is rarely performed after this stage unless the mothers health is in danger.

Abortion is a relatively safe procedure. Many women fear that the procedure may be painful and lead to complications. Less than 1% of women who have abortions experience a major complication such as a pelvic infection. There are myths that women that have abortions will have problems conceiving in the future. This is not true. There is no evidence of childbearing problems among women who have had a vacuum aspiration abortion, the most common procedure, within the first 12 weeks of pregnancy.

GETTING AN ABORTION

Once a woman has determined that she is pregnant and wishes to seek an abortion she should act quickly to terminate her pregnancy. Abortions that take place during the first trimester have less complications and are less expensive than abortions that take place later in the pregnancy. 88% of women who seek abortions have them in the first 12 weeks of pregnancy.

Abortions usually take place in clinics, doctor's offices or hospital facilities. The area that you live in will determine the cost and availability of getting the procedure done. In many large urban areas, abortions clinics are easily accessible. However, women that live in rural areas often have to travel hundreds of miles to obtain an abortion. Often when they reach the clinic, the cost may be much higher than the national average due to the fact that the clinic is the only one in the area that offers the procedure.

Once you have found a facility to perform the procedure, you should inquire about the cost of the procedure. In 1997, the cost of a non-hospital abortion with local anesthesia at 10 weeks of gestation ranged from $150 to $1,535 and the average amount paid was $316. The cost often depends on the area that you live in and the availability of other abortion providers in the area.

When you call for a quote, you will be asked how many weeks you are. If you can determine this on your own, they will provide a price quote. Before the procedure is done, most clinics will perform a vaginal scan ultrasound to properly date the pregnancy before the procedure is performed. 43% of all abortion facilities provide services only through the 12th week of pregnancy. If you find out that you are further along in your pregnancy than you calculated, you may have to re-consider your decision to have an abortion or find a facility that offers second trimester abortions.

INSURANCE AND OTHER PAYMENT METHODS

If you have insurance, your insurance provider may or may not pay for an induced abortion. It is best to ask the facility that is providing the procedure what type of insurance they accept. In addition, you should place a call to your insurance provider to make sure that your policy covers the procedure. If your insurance company does not cover the procedure you may have to pay cash for the procedure, or seek an alternative method of payment. Some states pay for abortions for women who cannot afford the procedure. 14% of abortions in this country are paid for by state funds.

It may also be wise to check with the facility to find out what type of payment methods they accept. Some abortion facilities do not accept checks, others only accept certain types of credit cards. Some facilities only accept money orders and don't take cash. It is important to find out this valuable information before you make the trip. Some clinics base the procedure on the number of weeks you are vs. the trimester. So it may be wise to have extra money available if it is determined you are further along than you calculated.

PARENTAL CONSENT

There is much to consider before getting an abortion . If you are a minor, certain states have parental consent laws. These laws vary from state to state. Parental consent laws require minors to have parental permission before receiving an abortion. Other states require parental notification. This only requires that parents be notified. All states allow the minor the opportunity to go before a judge if they do not want to involve their parents. This process is known as judicial bypass. The specifics of the laws vary from state to state. When you contact the facility to schedule your procedure they can inform you of the laws in your particular state.

*States that require parental consent or parental notification
AL, AR, DE, GA, IA, ID, IN, KS, KY, LA, MA, MD, MI, MN, MO, MS, NC, ND, NE, OH, OK, PA, RI, SC, SD, TN, TX, UT, VA,WI, WV, and WY.

*States that DO NOT require parental consent
AK, CA, CT, FL, HI, IL, MT, NV, NH, NJ, NM, OR, WA

*Current as of August 2004.

MANDATORY WAITING PERIODS
Another obstacle facing women wishing to obtain an abortion is waiting periods. Waiting periods are legally enforced waiting periods that a women must adhere to before getting an abortion. Mandatory waiting periods for abortions came into effect in 1992 following the Supreme Court decision in Planned Parenthood of Southeastern Pennsylvania v. Casey. This ruling enforced a mandatory 25 hour waiting period before an abortion can be performed. Currently 15 states require waiting periods.

In many instances a woman will have to come into the clinic for a counseling session and she will be required to return in 18-24 hours to have the procedure performed. This ruling can cause more strain in an already strenuous situation. 86% of the counties in the United States where a third of American women of childbearing age live, have no doctors trained, qualified, and willing to perform abortions.

If a woman has to travel a great distance or even out of state to get an abortion, the mandatory waiting period will cause her to have to spend more money on a hotel room and related travel expenses.

Mandatory waiting periods can make getting an abortion difficult for a woman who has to travel to get the procedure done. What if the woman has other children or a job that she can't get away from? Mandatory waiting periods may cause her to miss work or school and possibly cause her to make arrangements for childcare for her existing children—thus making her abortion more difficult to obtain. Time is of the essence when seeking an abortion. A day or two delay can cause a first trimester abortion to become a second trimester abortion—which is costlier and more risky.

INTAKE PROCEDURE

When you arrive at the abortion facility, you will be asked to fill out a short application. This form usually asks questions about your medical history and contact information in case of an emergency. Before you can get an abortion, it has to be determined that you are indeed pregnant and how far along in your pregnancy that you are. You will be given a pregnancy test and will undergo an ultrasound which will be used to accurately date your pregnancy. Your blood type will also be tested and your RH type will be noted.

PRE-ABORTION COUNSELING

The majority of abortion clinics offer some type of counseling before they perform your procedure. Depending on the facility, you may be offered one on one counseling or the counseling may take place in a group setting. If you are a minor you can opt to go into the counseling session by yourself or with your parents.

The one on one counseling will take place in a private area with you and an employee from the abortion clinic. The actual set up of the counseling session varies. Most of the time you will be asked if you desire an abortion and/or if you are seeking an abortion of your free will. If you are a minor they really try to determine whether or not you are being coerced into the procedure. Even if you come with a boyfriend, they will try to determine if it is your wish to get the abortion. No one can make you get an abortion if you don't want to. The clinic will not perform an abortion on you if you make it clear that this is not something that you want to do. After asking a few questions, they will explain the procedure to you.

Whether you are having a first trimester abortion or a second trimester abortion, they will explain the procedure and ask you if you have any questions. This counseling session is not intended to try to talk you out of getting the procedure or to dig deep into your personal business. The main focus is to make sure that you are getting the abortion of your own free will and that you are fully aware of the procedure.

If you are not getting your procedure done at the time of the counseling session due to a mandatory waiting period or due to scheduling reasons, the counselor will give you pre and post abortion instructions. This may include information about whether or not you can eat before the procedure, and any other special instructions. Most clinics require that women have an escort accompany them to the clinic to drive them home after the procedure. However, if you are having a first trimester abortion, you may be able to get around this if you agree to stay in the recovery area a little bit longer after your procedure or agree to make arrangements to take a cab.

At this time, they may also ask you if you have any birth control plans in place for the future. Depending on the clinic, they may give you birth control, such as a Depo-Provera shot or a pack of birth control pills. Other clinics may refer you to your regular OB/GYN or arrange birth control methods when you return for you follow up visit.

The group counseling is similar to the one on one counseling, except that it takes place within a group setting. You will be placed in a group with other women who are planning to have abortions. If you are a teen you may attend counseling with other women your age. Some clinics have certain days where they offer teen abortions. If you are not only with teens you will attend counseling with women of different ages. If the facility offers both first trimester and second trimester abortions, they may separate the counseling sessions and have women attend the session that applies to their length in their pregnancy.

In the group counseling session, the counselor will not put any one woman on the spot and ask her specific questions about her situation—in most cases. In the group counseling session, the counselor will explain the procedure and pre and post abortion procedures. At this time, they may ask the group which women are interested in obtaining birth control that day.

If the facility has a mandatory waiting period, the women will return the following day to have the procedure performed. If there is not a waiting period, the women usually will proceed to have the procedure performed after the counseling session.

In many instances, the facility will offer one on one counseling for the second trimester procedure. This is due to the fact that second trimester abortions are not as common as first trimester abortions and the woman has been pregnant longer and may need in depth counseling before actually having the procedure.

In some cases the woman seeking an abortion will be required to attend both a one on one and a group counseling session. The counseling aspect of the abortion procedure varies by clinic.

THE EARLY OPTION MEDICINAL ABORTION

The abortion pill or Mifeprex was approved by the FDA for abortions up to 7 weeks of gestation in the year 2000. You may also hear this pill referred to as RU-486. The introduction of this drug into American society gave women an alternative to a surgical abortion. Mifeprex allows an abortion to occur by blocking the hormones necessary to allow a pregnancy to continue. Mifeprex is used in combination with Misoprostol. Misoprostol is a prostaglandin that causes the uterus to contract. The drugs must be administered by a physician.

After you take the first dose of the drugs you will experience cramping and bleeding. The pregnancy will be terminated in 24 hours in most cases. A woman who decides on a medicinal abortion will usually have to visit her health care provider three times. When Mifeprex is used in conjunction with Misoprostol the results are 90% effective. If for some reason the medicinal abortion fails, which occurs in less than 10% of procedures, the woman will have to follow up with a surgical abortion.

Bleeding and cramping are a normal part of the procedure. Some side effects include headaches, nausea, vomiting, diarrhea, dizziness, and fatigue. Not all women will experience these side effects. If any of the side effects become severe you should contact the doctors office where you had the procedure performed immediately. Medicinal abortions have been performed in Europe for years and the procedure is popular. The procedure is gaining in popularity in the United States as more abortion facilities begin to offer medicinal abortions.

In November of 2004, the United States FDA strengthened the warning label for the drug Mifeprex. The new warning labels will warn doctors about how the drug should not be used in ectopic pregnancy and the label will warn doctors and patients of the possible risk of infection and heavy bleeding. Although, complications with Mifeprex are rare, the FDA wants people to be warned.

THE ABORTION PROCEDURE –FIRST TRIMESTER

The first trimester abortion procedure is far less evasive and lengthy as the second trimester abortion procedure. You will be wearing a hospital gown and be required to lay down and place your feet in stirrups. The doctor performing the procedure and a nurse will be in attendance. Prior to the procedure you may be given the option to choose the type of anesthesia that you would prefer. Some clinics offer general (asleep) anesthesia for first trimester abortions. This type of anesthesia may cost more. Other anesthesia types are twilight (conscious) or local (numb the area, awake). Patients receiving anesthesia will be closely monitored with special attention given to blood pressure and vital signs. A gynecologist with special expertise in abortions performs the procedure by a method known as vacuum aspiration. If you are 10 weeks or less, and if available, you may be given your abortion by manual aspiration. This involves the use of a specially designed syringe to apply suction.

If manual aspiration is not available or if you are 12 weeks or less, your abortion may be performed by a vacuum machine. This is the most common first trimester abortion procedure. This method involves the use of a hollow tube that is attached by tubing to a bottle and a pump, which provides a gentle vacuum. The tube, which is called a Cannula is passed into the uterus, the pump is turned on, and the tissue is gently removed from the uterus. If all of the tissues are not removed you may be given a D&C. D&C is short for dilation and cutterage and it involves removing any remaining tissues after the aspiration procedure.

The procedure lasts anywhere from 7-15 minutes. After the procedure, the tissues removed will be examined to make sure that the abortion was complete. Some clinics take it a step further and also provide a post abortion ultrasound. First-trimester therapeutic surgical abortions are safe and effective and have few complications. About 90% of all abortions are done in the first trimester of pregnancy.

THE SECOND TRIMESTER ABORTION
The second trimester abortion is a two step procedure in most cases, but increasingly many clinics are offering safe second trimester abortions in a one step setting. However, the majority of abortion clinics still perform second trimester abortions in two steps.

Due to the fact that the pregnancy has progressed, you will have to be dilated before the procedure can be performed. Small sticks known as laminara or some other type of synthetic dilator will be inserted into the cervix to help open the cervix. Opening the cervix protects the cervix during the procedure and allows the instruments to not harm the cervix during the procedure. Once the artificial dilators are inserted, the woman will leave the facility and return in 18-24 hours to have the procedure performed.

Similar to the first trimester abortion, you will be wearing a hospital type gown and be required to lie on a table with your feet in stirrups. Your vital signs will be monitored and you will be given anesthesia. Depending on how many weeks you are and your preference, you may be given a general (asleep) anesthesia versus an awake form of anesthesia. If you are given general anesthesia you will only given enough to last during the time needed to complete the procedure and you will wake up shortly after the procedure.

The second trimester abortion involves getting a D&E. D&E is short for a procedure known as dilation and evacuation. This procedure is similar to a D&C, but it involves several methods. A D&E can consist of a combination of vacuum aspiration, D&C, and the use of surgical instruments such as forceps. The D&E procedure usually lasts 30 minutes.

After the procedure, tissues are examined and an ultrasound may also be performed to ensure that the abortion process was complete.

RECOVERY
The recovery period after an abortion is very important. The abortion facility will have to monitor you and your bleeding after the procedure. The main things that they will be monitoring you for are heavy bleeding and fevers. Heavy bleeding can indicate a serious condition and a fever can be a sign of infection. You will be asked to lie down and they will give you a light snack and something to drink. This may consist of graham crackers or saltines and juice. You will be given post-operative medications and any antibiotics you will need to take. If you like, they may allow the person who accompanied you to the clinic to come and see you in the recovery area.

For first trimester abortions they may require you to stay in the recovery area for 45 minutes to an hour. For second trimester abortions you will most likely have to remain at the facility for several hours after your procedure.

Before leaving the clinic, they will once again explain after care procedures. They may schedule a follow up appointment at that facility or you may schedule a follow up visit with your regular doctor at a later date. They will also provide you with any birth control that you may have requested.

HOW YOU WILL FEEL AFTERWARDS
Women report different feelings after an abortion. Some women experience only light cramps similar to menstrual cramps. Others report severe cramping. Where some women bleed only for a few days after the procedure, others may bleed for several weeks after the procedure. No one can predict and tell you how you will feel

emotionally and physically after the procedure. The range of emotions experienced varies from woman to woman. If you feel severely depressed or even that you just need to talk to someone, there are many places out there that can offer you the post abortion counseling that you need.

AFTER CARE

After your abortion you will be released from the clinic. The clinic may provide you with antibiotics or a prescription for antibiotics. It is important that you take all of the medication given to you. You will also be provided with after care instructions. It is important to follow these directions very carefully. Failure to follow the instructions may lead to an infection or another pregnancy. Common after care instructions include:

- No bathing
- No douching
- No insertion of any medications or tampons in the vagina
- No sexual intercourse for 1-2 weeks.

THE FOLLOW UP VISIT

2-3 weeks after your abortion you will be attending a follow up visit with your regular physician or at the facility that performed your abortion. At this time a pelvic exam will be administered and you will also be given a pregnancy test . It is very important that you don't skip the follow-up visit. Even if you feel 100% fine, the follow-up visit is a necessity. The reason that a pregnancy test is administered is to guarantee a negative result.

The doctor may ask you how your current method of birth control is working and may permit you to have sex again. Depending on the procedure you had, you may have been required to wait one or two weeks before resuming sexual intercourse.

An induced abortion rarely affects your future fertility. Most women who have abortions go on to have children if they so desire. It is important to use a reliable method of birth control following your procedure because you will be able to conceive soon after.

Some abortion facilities offer counseling at the follow up visit.

Sandra, age 16   **Here Again**

"Unfortunately, I have been here before. At the clinic—again. I was 13 the first time I got pregnant. My mom found out and brought me here. I was so freaked out after the whole thing I swore I would never have sex again. I started taking the pill but was too afraid the pill would make me fat. I stopped taking the pill and sophomore year I found myself pregnant again. I don't want to have a baby right now. I want to finish school, go to college, do something. Yes, I know I have heard it all before, you can do it all and be a mom, but the truth is I don't want to be a mom right now and the guy that got me pregnant is a jerk. After this abortion my mom is going to see if I am old enough for an IUD or she might get me the birth control shot."

Amber, age 22   **Mr. Right Turned Out To Be Mr. Wrong**

"I had been dating Eric for 3 years when I got pregnant. I was a senior in college and he had just graduated. I was living in Virginia and he was attending law school in North Carolina. We really only had time to see each other on altering weekends. We had been sexually active for our entire relationship. With him away most of the time I stopped using the pill. We never used condoms because we were in a monogamous relationship. One particular weekend we had sex and I told him to "pull out," but he didn't.

I considered keeping the baby. The timing was poor, but we had talked of marriage in the past. I thought we would just change our plans and get married sooner. When I told Eric I was pregnant he totally flipped. He told me we were "too young," and that he had "just started law school," and that I was "trying to trap him and tie him down." I couldn't believe he said those things to me. I was devastated and thought about having the baby on my own. But then I talked to my parents and friends and decided that not having the baby would be best. There were so many things I wanted to do in life, and having a baby at that moment, and doing it on my own, would have changed everything in my life.

We agreed on me having an abortion and Eric was a jerk about it. He didn't even come to take me to get the procedure. He paid for it, but get this—he had one of his frat brothers drop the money off at my door one evening.

After the abortion I was depressed. It didn't hurt too bad and the procedure went rather quickly. I was sad because a part of me wanted to keep the baby. I was also sad because I couldn't believe how fast Eric changed on me. After the abortion Eric and I never talked again. Now I am 26 years old and happily married to a wonderful man with a baby on the way. All I can say is everything happens for a reason."

Caitlin, age 16　　　　　**The Day I Cut Class**

"I was raised in Albany, New York. My home life was stable. I had two parents who adored me and a wonderful little brother. When I started high school, I don't know if I was rebelling or what, but my best friend Rachel and I really got into the whole "goth" thing. I dyed my blonde hair jet black and purple, and I pierced my tongue, lip and eye brow. I only wore black and my parents hated it. They always told me I needed counseling, but at the same time, my grades didn't drop so they couldn't complain too much. They chalked it up as me going through a phase.

One day sophomore year, Rachel and I cut class and decided to hang out at my friend Frankie's house. He was goth too. We listened to music and had a couple of drinks. There was a guy at the house named Chad. He was 24, goth, and he was cute. Rachel and I had never seen him before, but since he was Frankie's friend he was cool. We all did some "E" that day, but it was no big deal because we had done "E" before.

Rachel and Frankie left to go to the grocery store to get something or other. I was out of it from the alcohol and the "E", but I was well aware of what was going on. Chad asked me to come in Frankie's bedroom and listen to a CD that they had made. I followed him into the bedroom. Once we got in there he held me down on the bed and started to pull down my pants. I begged him to stop and he grabbed my breast and stuck his tongue in my mouth. He raped me for what seemed like hours, but was in all actuality only about 20 minutes. I didn't scream because no one was in the house. When he heard Rachel and Frankie return from the store he stopped.

I didn't report the rape to the authorities because I had been drinking and using drugs and I thought no one would believe me. About a month later, I discovered I was pregnant. I was 15 years old, and I was in no way ready to become a parent. I confided in my mother that I was pregnant and we made arrangements for me to have an abortion. I kept the rape a secret, and I did not reveal to her who the father of the child was.

I didn't have an abortion just because I conceived during a rape. I was young and wasn't ready to be a parent. I do not feel guilty about having the abortion and I don't believe I bear any emotional scars from the abortion. However, I feel that I am still recovering from the emotional trauma of the rape."

Cynthia, age 15   **A game with real life consequences**

"One month I had a period and the next month I didn't. I was 12 years old and I didn't think anything of it. I told my mom, who never would have imagined that I was pregnant. She called our family doctor who advised her that sometimes young women have irregular menstrual cycles.

I guess I should start at the beginning. My name is Cynthia and when I was 12 years old I got pregnant. I didn't know I had sex. I thought I was still a virgin. So how did I end up pregnant?

At my cousin Sheri's 14th Halloween party, we played a game of truth or dare. We were just having a good time playing games and eating candy and pizza. I had on a short skirt and a tight shirt. I was the youngest girl at the party. My breasts were just starting to grow in. Some of the kids at the party dared me to go into the closet with a boy named Vincent and to let him stick his thing in me for one minute.

I wanted to be like the older girls who had been doing wild dares all night. I followed Vincent, who was 14, into the closet. Everyone wanted to watch! They said they wanted to make sure we did it. I said, "Can you please close the door?" They closed the closet door and everyone started to mock me, "Can you please close the door."

In the closet I lifted up my skirt and kept my panties on. Vincent pulled down his pants and tried to put his thing in me. I don't even know if he got it in all the way. Before I knew it, my panties were all wet and the group outside opened the door and started pointing and laughing. That Monday, everyone at school teased me for going in the closet with Vincent.

My period stopped coming and I didn't think anything about it. I didn't know I was pregnant. My breasts grew bigger and my hips got bigger. I was in 7th grade and more boys started to like me. My mom figured it was puberty, until one day my mother and I were at Sears trying on clothes and she looked at my stomach. She asked me if I was pregnant and I said, "No."

Soon after my mother took me to the doctor and discovered I was pregnant. I wasn't just a little pregnant. I was real pregnant. I was about 17 ½ weeks. My mother pressured me about who I was having sex with, and I told her I hadn't had sex with anyone. I didn't know anything about being pregnant. My family found out and my cousin told my mom about the Halloween party. I didn't have a choice, my mother was taking me to get an abortion. I didn't know what I wanted, but then again I was a baby myself.

The first clinic we went to didn't take patients under 13 years of age, due to the fact that their body is still developing and so on. Then all of the other clinics in our area only offered first trimester abortions. My mother ended up taking me to another state to get an abortion. I remember us being turned away by so many clinics due to my age. When we finally found a clinic, it was costly, $1400. That was a lot of money and I knew my mom didn't have any money to spare. She took a cash advance off of her credit card to pay for the procedure.

At the clinic I was counseled, and when I found out what an abortion was, I changed my mind. I didn't want to have one. I wanted to keep the baby. My mother was not hearing me though, and since she was my guardian, she pretty much ran the situation.

After the abortion, I remember waking up after the procedure and thrashing my body all about and I fell off of the recovery room table. I was screaming and crying. I was having horrible cramps and I felt bad because the baby I just found out about a few days earlier was gone. I cried the whole time in the recovery room and the whole ride home. I was bleeding so much, and so depressed that my mom let me stay home a whole week from school.

It was a bad situation, but now that I am older I realize that my mom did the right thing for me at the time. I'm a freshman in high school, and very active in school. I still consider myself a virgin because that incident was so strange. I love my mom and I'm glad that she did what she did for me. I couldn't imagine being someone's parent right now. Everything worked out for me thanks to her persistence and love for me."

Zena, age 21   Just Not Ready
"I have a medical condition/disease that I do not want to state. People with this condition have gone on to have very healthy babies. I have been ill for much of my childhood and adult life. I knew how not to get pregnant, but I was very careless with the pill. When faced with an unplanned pregnancy, I considered having the baby. When I discussed the health risks, I opted to have an abortion. Some people might say, "Oh you are wrong for having an abortion." At 21, I was just starting my life and didn't want to take that chance." If abortion was not legal, I would have had to take the risk no matter what. For the record, I do want to have children one day. I want to wait until I am married and am financially stable. At that time, I think I will be mentally prepared to take the risk."

Chapter 7- Adoption—The Option

It may be a scary thing to consider going through nine months of pregnancy only to give the child to another family to raise. Adoption is an option that many women facing unplanned pregnancies turn to. These women are brave enough to realize that they may not have the resources to raise a child on their own, and at the same time they may also not believe in abortion or not want to have the procedure. Adoption as an option can be a win/win situation but as with having a child or terminating a pregnancy there is an emotional aspect involved with giving a child up for adoption.

ADOPTION

Adoption is the act of giving your child to another family to raise. Adoption is a legal act, and by choosing adoption you will permanently give your child to another family to raise. If you choose adoption, there are many people and organizations that can help you proceed with your decision. Adoption does not have to be a scary thing. It can be a loving choice for you and your child. There are several types of adoption.

OPEN ADOPTION

An open adoption is one where the birth parents and the adoptive parents have knowledge of one another and may have an open line of communication. Often times the birth mother will interview prospective adoptive parents. If the two agree on an open adoption, they may decide on a level of contact to continue after the birth of the child. Sometimes the birth mother and the adoptive parents will agree that the adoptive parents send pictures. The level of openness is dependent on the parties involved. Any type of open adoption agreement should be legally binding and a lawyer should be involved.

If you agree to enter into an open adoption arrangement, realize that the adoptive parents will legally be the child's parents. If the adopted parents don't do something that you like as far as raising the child you can't petition the court for visitation or demand that they do things the way that you want them to be done.

There are varying degrees of open adoption. A type of adoption that falls into the open adoption category is semi-open adoption. In this type of adoption the birth parents and adoptive parents may meet to form an agreement as to the degree of future contact. This may entail the frequency that pictures be sent or detail a chance to meet the child at a future date. It is important to remember that open adoption is not a shared custody agreement. The birth parents still terminate all parental rights.

CLOSED ADOPTION
A closed adoption severs all communication between the birth parents and the adoptive parents. The birth parents and adoptive parents know very little information, if any, about each other. The records remain sealed.

KINSHIP ADOPTION
A kinship adoption is an adoption that takes place when a grandparent, aunt, uncle, other extended family member adopts a child. This type of adoption has been happening for years. If you are considering a kinship adoption, it is best to get a lawyer involved to make sure that all legal aspects are covered.

CONFIDENTIAL ADOPTION
In a confidential adoption, the birth parents and the adoptive parents do not know each others identity. The only information that the prospective adoptive parents are given about you and the birth father is your medical history.

PRIVATE ADOPTION
A private adoption is one that does not go through an adoption agency. This type of adoption is also referred to as independent adoption sometimes. A private adoption is one where the birth

mother has no contact with the birth parents after the adoption. The birth mother can view profiles of prospective birth parents and choose a family for her child. The birth parents and the prospective adoptive parents work through a licensee. The birth parents will have to sign a consent form to release the child to the adoptive family. Although a consent form is signed, the birth parents will have a window in time in which they can change their mind and get their child back. The time allowed for reversing a private adoption varies from state to state.

Sometimes there are degrees of contact with a private adoption. Often times the birth parents and the adoptive parents will set up an agreement with a lawyer, third party to send non identifying pictures to the birth parents.

Depending on your adoption situation, the prospective parents or the adoption agency may pay for your prenatal care and delivery if you do not have insurance. Research any agency that you plan to deal with carefully. If they ever ask you for money, look elsewhere. The birth mother should not have to pay a listing fee or any type of fees when they choose to place their child up for adoption.

CONSENT
Whether you are married or single, to place your child up for adoption, you and the birth father will have to sign a document terminating parental rights. A biological father, or alleged biological father has to consent to adoption if he has been notified that he is the father and has taken steps to support the child.

A putative father is the alleged father of a child born out of wedlock. A putative father has no legal rights to a child until he has taken action to establish paternity. He must establish paternity to receive notice of adoption proceedings or to contest an adoption.

Different states have different laws regarding putative fathers rights in regards to adoption. When you begin the adoption process you will be informed of the steps you need to take in regards to the child's father and the adoption process.

GETTING STARTED WITH THE ADOPTION PROCESS

If you have chosen or are leaning in the direction of adoption it is important to start planning your child's adoption early in your pregnancy. Part of the planning includes educating yourself on the adoption process and the adoption laws in your state. The resources below can assist you in getting started with the adoption process.

ADOPTION RESOURCES

National Adoption Information Clearinghouse

The National Adoption Information Clearinghouse is a resource with a wealth of information on adoption. The Clearinghouse is a service of Children's Bureau, Administration on Children, Youth and Families, Administration for Children and Families, Department of Health and Human Services. Their services for birth mothers are free. This should be your first step when considering adoption versus just jumping on the Internet. They are not an adoption agency but they can provide you with educational materials about adoption. They can also give you listings for adoption agencies and Pregnancy Centers in your area that can assist with your adoption.

You can visit them on the web at:
http://naic.acf.hhs.gov/

Pregnancy Centers

Pregnancy Centers provide free, confidential services to pregnant women. They not only provide free pregnancy testing and counseling, but they also provide adoption support and assistance. Many Pregnancy Centers also are licensed adoption agencies.

Adoption Agencies

An adoption agency is a licensed agency that provides services to birth parents and adoptive parents. Adoption agencies can be non-profit, for profit, religious based, public or private. When choosing an agency, make sure that the agency is licensed. If they ask you for any money, this can be a red flag. The birth mother should not have to pay any money, such as for a listing fee, when she is considering adoption.

Health Department or Social Services
If you contact your local health department they can refer you to the appropriate state agency that can assist you with your adoption.

Newspaper advertisements, flyers, Internet web sites from couples
Beware. As infertility is seemingly on the rise, there are more couples desperate to adopt children. They will post pictures around town, post advertisements in newspapers and even create web pages to make themselves seem appealing as prospective adoptive parents. As stated previously, get a lawyer if you plan on pursuing an adoption lead that you find out about outside of an agency.

PROTECT YOURSELF
It is important that you have an attorney or an advocate that is knowledgeable about the adoption process that will represent you and make sure that your wishes are being followed and that the best interest of you and your child are primary. Even if your resources are low, you may be able to find an adoption attorney.

FUTURE CONTACT
You may decide that you want to find your child one day when they become an adult or vice versa your child may decide to seek you one day. If you choose a confidential adoption, there may be ways for you to leave information about yourself to help your child locate you in the future. Many states have set up adoption registries. The way that the registries work is that you submit information about yourself and the birth of the child to the registry. You will leave your phone number and address with the registry. If the child decides to search for you in the future and the

information that they have regarding their birth matches up with the information provided by you, the registry will release your information to the child.

Another method is that some adoption agencies and lawyers who handle adoptions will keep a letter in the child's file that has specific information about you and how to contact you. Not all attorneys and agencies will agree to this in a confidential adoption, so you may wish to choose an agency that will follow your wishes. Remember, this is your child and you have rights on how you want your adoption to be carried through.

STORIES OF ADOPTION

Shandi, age 15   Scared and Afraid
"When I became pregnant I was scared and afraid. I knew that I did not want to become a mother. I wanted to stay in school. None of my friends had babies. My family arranged for an open adoption. My boyfriends family also felt that adoption was the best alternative. A church family adopted my baby. They came to get the baby when she was born. I don't feel bad or miss the baby. I am glad they were there to take the baby. I learned a powerful lesson about life. I am still sexually active with my boyfriend but much more careful now."

Sue, Age 28   The Child My Family Will Never Know
"I came to the United States on a student visa to study medicine. I came to the US from Japan. I am the youngest child of my parents and I have 3 older brothers. It was difficult for me to convince my parents to send me to the US to continue my education. They felt like there were plenty of good schools in Japan and being the only female, they weren't quite sure I needed to become a doctor.

I desperately wanted to prove them wrong and succeed. During my last year of medical school, I was dating another medical student named Robert. Unexpectedly, I became pregnant. We were not ready to be parents.

We decided that we would place the child up for adoption. Initially, when I contacted adoption agencies, they told me that they may have a hard time placing a Japanese child, but when they found out the father was white, they said that may help me find an adoptive family easier.

Robert and I screened every family carefully and we were lucky enough to find an Asian woman and a white male who were looking for a bi-racial child. This was wonderful because I was concerned about my child being raised by 100% non-Asian parents.

It was hard for me to sign away the baby boy Robert and I had, but it was for the best. I finished my residency after medical school and only plan on staying in the United States for a few more years. I plan to return to Japan permanently to be near my family.

My family and I are very close, yet I never told them about the child I gave birth to. I feel bad because my family is so close and it is hard to imagine that part of my family blood line is out there and will never know us."

Tarnisha, age 22   Know Your Rights!

"If you are considering giving your child up for adoption, know your rights! I became pregnant my senior year of high school. My aunt and were like the best of friends. She is 12 years older than me, so we were more like sisters than aunt and niece. When she found out I was pregnant with a little girl, she begged to adopt my baby. She had always wanted a girl and all of her other children were boys.

I went away to college after the baby was born. The baby, a little girl named Shelly, fit in perfect with my aunt's family. Although my aunt raised the child since birth, we never signed any paperwork other than a simple guardianship form for medical care.

To make a long story short, when I graduated and started working in my field as a biochemist, my aunt became very jealous of my $50,000 a year salary. Her exact words were, "That's too much money for one person with no responsibilities other than rent and a car note." She went as far as to tell me that I owed her child support. How would I owe her child support if she was the adoptive mother? Our relationship quickly soured and my aunt even tried to take me to court over the money. She also started telling people the only agreement was that she keep Shelly until I finished school. My aunt even went as far as to tell me to, "Come and get your daughter." By this time, Shelly was 5. My then boyfriend knew nothing about me having given birth to a child, so I had to explain Shelly to him. I also had to change my schedule at work to accommodate my new state of motherhood.

Shelly only knew me as Auntie Tarnisha and it was devastating for her to be taken away from the only mother that she had ever known and her brothers. My aunt and I lived in separate states so I only saw Shelly around the holidays. The relationship between my aunt and me is destroyed. If you are considering family adoption, or any type of adoption, make sure that everything is legal!"

Nancy, age 18- Foster care, a baby and a young girl without a home

"When I was 15 years old, my life was in turmoil to say the least. I never knew my father. My mother was a drug addict who died of AIDS when I was 13 years old. I was placed in the custody of my aunt who was very strict. I couldn't take it and I ran away to live on the streets. My aunt could not care for me and was determined not to let me slip away, so she made sure that I was placed in foster care. I soon became a ward of the state. I bounced from foster home to foster home.

I had a boyfriend named Ted. I would hide out at his house instead of going to school and we would drink and have sex. My foster mother suspected I was pregnant and took me to the doctor. I was 4 ½ months pregnant when I found out I was pregnant. I actually considered keeping the baby. When I told Ted, he told me that I was a "runaway, throw-away slut" and that the baby probably wasn't his.

My foster mother was in "too deep," she said. She turned me back over to the court system. They placed me in a home for girls. Since I was a ward of the state, they told me that I would either have to stay in the girls home, a maternity shelter or find a foster parent that was willing to take me and my baby. I didn't have anything. I felt like the best thing would be to place the child up for adoption.

I learned a little bit about the birth parents, their careers and about their other kids and decided to go the adoption route. I gave birth to a healthy baby girl at 8 months and she was adopted shortly after. The adoption was a closed adoption.

Three years later, a part of me really regrets my decision. Now I am 18, I finished my GED and I have my own apartment. I work and I am planning to go to city college. I wish that more people would have taken an interest in me and helped me see that I could have kept my baby and been alright. But I hope that she has a nice life now."

Diane, age 22   **I never wanted to even look at the baby**

"My boyfriend and I were together for 3 years before we had our first child. Our son Abe meant the world to us. After Abe was born, my boyfriend started drinking more and we argued more than ever. When our son was two years old I found out that I was pregnant again. We immediately knew that we were not ready for more kids. I had planned on having an abortion but time slipped away and I didn't have the money for the more costly second trimester procedure. We decided to give the baby up for adoption.

I did not become attached to this baby. I tried to ignore the babies kicks and I didn't even want to look at the ultrasound picture. When my boyfriend found out the baby was another boy he started having second thoughts.

My mind was made up. When I went into labor, I didn't even pack a bag for the new baby. When I gave birth, I told the doctor I didn't even want to see the baby. After the baby was born they took him straight to the nursery. Before I was discharged I signed the adoption papers.

I never did see the baby. It may sound cold hearted that I never saw the baby, but I knew I would just melt. I had to stay strong to follow through with my decision."

CHAPTER 8-Desperate Acts-Safe Haven Laws

Child abandonment should never be considered a viable option when faced with an unplanned pregnancy. Child abandonment of newborns has only slightly risen over the past decade, but cases are receiving more media attention than they have in the past. Desperation has driven young mothers to dispose of their newborn infants in toilets and garbage cans. Many of these mothers managed to conceal their pregnancy and were full term at the time they delivered. It is terrible that things like this happen with all of the resources available for young women facing unplanned pregnancies but it does happen. These young women are often motivated by fear and desperation. In an effort to curb infanticide and the reckless disposal of new born babies, a handful of states have enacted Safe Haven laws.

Leslie Harris shocked the film industry in 1993 with the release of her independent film, *Just Another Girl on The IRT*. The film won a special Jury Prize at the 1993 Sundance Film Festival and was distributed by Miramax.

The film tells the story of a teenage girl named Chantel Mitchell who had high hopes and aspirations for the future. Raised in the projects of New York by poor working class parents, Chantel had her sites set on graduating from high school a year early and heading to college. Chantel's plans were sidetracked when she finds herself pregnant. Chantel acts in a behavior that is typical of many young women facing an unplanned pregnancy. She is scared, and she tries to push her pregnancy to the back of her mind. Chantel hides her pregnancy, only revealing it to her boyfriend and a clinic worker. Her boyfriend pressures her to have an abortion and he even goes as far to give Chantel the money for the procedure. Chantel uses the money to go on a shopping spree with her friend. Chantel never followed through with the abortion.

With no prenatal care, Chantel goes into premature labor at 29 weeks. With her boyfriends assistance, they wrap the baby in a plastic bag and dispose of the baby outside in a trash dumpster.

However, second thoughts prevent them from actually following through.

Sadly, many women feel so desperate that they simply feel the urge to "get rid of the baby." Sometimes they feel so desperate that they don't care about the safety or the well being of the infant, as long as the child is gone they feel as if their problem will be solved. They don't think about the well being of the child or the possible legal problems that they can face from law enforcement if they commit a crime.

Abandonment or infanticide should never be considered an option when there are so many safe options for women facing unwanted pregnancy. Infanticide is the murder of an infant born alive. The Amy Grossburg and Brian Peterson Case gained national attention in 1996 when the two high school sweethearts were suspected of killing their newborn son and leaving the infant in a motel trash dumpster. Grossburg had managed to conceal her pregnancy from her family and gave birth to a healthy full term boy. The couple later pled guilty to manslaughter charges and served less than three years in prison.

Another infanticide case that drew national attention was the case of New Jersey V Melissa Drexler, a case often referred to as "The Prom Mom" case. Eighteen year old Melissa Drexler concealed her pregnancy from her family, friends, and even the suspected child's father—her 19 year old prom date. On the morning of her prom, the 130 pound teens water broke. Soon after arriving at the prom, Melissa experienced cramping and went into the bathroom where she delivered a full term baby boy. After strangling the infant and placing him in numerous garbage bags, Melissa threw the infant in a garbage can and returned to the prom.

Melissa initially was to face murder charges, but after pleading guilty to a lesser charge she read the following statement in court:

"I knew I was pregnant. I concealed the pregnancy from everyone. On the morning of the prom my water broke. While I was in the car on the way to the prom, I began to have cramps. I went to the prom and I went into the bathroom and delivered the baby. The baby was born alive. I knowingly took the baby out the toilet and wrapped a series of garbage bags around the baby. I then placed the baby in another garbage bag, knotted it closed and threw it in the trash can. I was aware of what I was doing at the time when I placed the baby in the bag. And I was further aware that what I did would most certainly result in the death of the baby."

In 1998, Melissa Drexler was sentenced to 15 years in prison. She was released in 2001 after serving nearly 4 years in prison. The infanticide cases mentioned are tragic and the worst possible result of infant abandonment.

Forty-five states have enacted a very controversial law that allows mothers the opportunity to leave their newborn infants at so called "safe havens" with no questions asked and facing no criminal charges, as long as the infants are healthy. Although the actual type of "safe haven" varies from state to state, most of the states that support this legislation allow the mothers to leave the newborns at police stations, fire stations, hospitals or other approved locations. The laws also vary from state to state, however most laws require that the child be less than 30 days old and of good health with no signs of abuse. The thirty day rule is not the norm. Most states require the child to be less than one week old so it is important that you know the legislation in your state if you ever feel this desperate. Most of the states say that the mother is immune from prosecution if the child is left in good health with no signs of abuse. Texas was the first state to sign the "Baby Moses" legislation under then Governor George W. Bush in 1999.

Many argue that Safe Haven legislation is telling the mother that it is okay to just abandon her child. However, with child abandonment and infanticide taking place anyway, Safe Haven legislation offers a safe alternative for the extremely desperate birth mother.

After the infants are left at Safe Havens, they are first given physical examinations to determine whether they are in good health. Then depending on the state, most of the children are either placed in foster care or immediately placed for adoption.

Another criticism of Safe Haven legislation is that adoption advocates feel that Safe Haven laws prevent the child from ever learning anything about their genealogy or medical history if need be. Also, what about the father? Are the fathers rights protected if a mother drops off a baby at a Safe Haven approved location?

Giving birth is a serious medical procedure. No young woman should plan to give birth in secrete. Just because someone else was able to give birth alone and survive without complications, you would put yourself and your baby at great risk if you decided to try to go it alone and give birth in secrecy. Many complications can arise during child birth which is why it is very important to give birth in a hospital or a setting where there are midwives or doulas present.

If you are planning on giving your child up for adoption, the Safe Haven option shouldn't be looked at as a cheap and easy adoption. Safe Haven legislation is only meant to help the most desperate of mothers. With a traditional adoption you have certain rights that you may not have if you simply abandon your child at a Safe Haven location. Also, Safe Haven shouldn't be looked at as an option of not wanting anyone to know that you had a baby. If you truly want to keep your pregnancy and birth of your child a secret, there are adoption agencies that can assist you with this process.

A STORY OF ABANDONMENT

Bethany, Age 15

The summer after 8th grade I got pregnant. I know how I got pregnant. I had sex and didn't use protection. I wanted to have a baby. My boyfriend Lamont was 16 years old and he lived in Englewood and I stayed out in Santa Ana. My mother had a good job and a Section 8 apartment so we had left Englewood but I still took the bus out there to visit my old neighborhood.

I didn't really fit in with the kids in my neighborhood in Santa Ana and that really drew me to keep going back to Englewood and Lamont. I enjoyed having sex with him. I never took a pregnancy test but I knew I was pregnant. By Thanksgiving time I couldn't even fit my jeans anymore. I told Lamont and he said his sister would take care of the baby until we were able to get an apartment.

One Friday evening when I was in Englewood, I went into labor in the middle of the night. I had the baby on Lamont's grandmothers bathroom floor. Afterwards, we went to the hospital to get checked out and I gave them Lamont sisters name and used her Medicaid card. They gave us both a clean bill of health and discharged us. Even though the baby was early, she was big enough to go home.

I told Lamont I had to go home to get some clothes for the baby and to explain to my mama what happened. I couldn't just show up at her door with a baby. Lamont understood and we took the baby over to his sisters apartment with a promise that we would be back the next day to pick up the baby.

When I got home, I couldn't tell mama. I had just turned 14 and I knew she would be disappointed so I just didn't say anything. I went to school like everything was normal. I had managed to carry the baby up until 34 weeks without my mother noticing I was pregnant because I wore baggy clothes. Not being pregnant felt so good.

Three days later Lamont started calling like crazy. I didn't return his calls. I convinced my mother that he was harassing me and she changed the phone number. Lamont had never been to my home in Santa Ana so I thought I could just make a clean break and never see him or the baby again and just go about my life.

Three weeks passed and I thought I was home free. I had met some new friends and a new guy and was finally starting to enjoy my freshman year. One evening as I was sitting on the couch, the doorbell rang. It was Lamont, his sister, and an Orange County Sheriff.

I was in a lot of mess. There were many unanswered questions and mama was devastated. After a lot of legal drama, my mother was awarded full custody of the baby girl who I named Trisha. I didn't want to be a mother. I couldn't hang out, I had no time for me.

Chapter 9- Birth Control For The Future

CONTRACEPTION

After your pregnancy has ended, whether you continued your pregnancy to term or you terminated your pregnancy, you may initially think that you won't have sex again for a very long time. Your body will heal and you will most likely engage in sexual activity again in your lifetime.

Rather than just swearing that you will never have sex again, (although it is your right to pursue abstinence), it's better to plan ahead for your next sexual encounter. If you are prepared, you can take the necessary steps to prevent another unplanned pregnancy.

Abstinence
Abstinence is the act of refraining from sexual intercourse. Abstinence is the safest method of birth control. Refraining from sexual intercourse will definitely eliminate any chance of becoming pregnant. However, some people may find abstinence a difficult method of birth control and others may not consider it at all. If you do consider abstinence or another form of abstinence called "Second Virginity" there are many support groups that will help you with your decision.

The Birth Control Pill
The birth control pill is the most popular reversible birth control method on the market. Birth control pills are oral hormones that when taken daily prevent pregnancy. The pills come in packs of 21 or 28 pills. When used daily without user error, the Pill is 95% effective. The pill does have some added benefits such as reduced menstrual bleeding and cramps and a reduction to the risk of ovarian cancer. The Pill is available from a doctor via prescription. Women who smoke or have heart conditions should not consider taking the pill. These women face an increased risk of heart attacks and blood clots. The Pill has been around since the 1960's and is a highly effective choice for birth control. The Pill is

reversible and women can conceive after cessation of Pill use. The Pill is most effective when used daily around the same time.

Possible Side Effects
- Side effects can include weight gain, headaches and moodiness

Depo-Provera

Depo-Provera is commonly known as "The Birth Control Shot." Depo-Provera is a form of birth control administered via a shot that will prevent pregnancy for three months at a time. If Depo-Provera is a woman's choice for birth control, she will only have to worry about birth control 4 times a year. Depo-Provera prevents pregnancy by releasing a hormone similar to progesterone. The popularity of Depo-Provera grew in the 1990's. Depo-Provera can be administered by a doctor, nurse or health care professional. Depo-Provera is reversible and it is 99% effective when preventing pregnancy.

Possible Side Effects
- Weight gain
- Irregularity or cessation of menstrual cycles

Male Condoms
Condoms are a popular form of contraceptive. A woman doesn't have to alter her body with hormones, male condoms place the responsibility of birth control on the male sex partner. Condoms are a barrier method of birth control, which means they prevent sperm from entering the vaginal canal. They are 86% effective and inexpensive, costing about .25 cents to .50 cents each. To increase the effectiveness of condoms, they should be used in conjunction with spermicide.

Common Complaints
- Can tear or slip off
- Effectiveness based on using the condom every time sexual intercourse takes place
- Some men complain of decrease in sexual pleasure

Female Condom
The female condom is available but has not gained as much popularity as the male condom. The female condom is more expensive. They average about $3 each. The female condom is worn inside of the vagina and its edges cover the woman's genitalia. Like the male condom, the female condom is available at drug stores without a prescription.

Common Complaints
- Often difficult to use and can slip during sexual activity

Inter Uterine Device (IUD)
An IUD is a small device implanted into the uterus to prevent pregnancy. The IUD is a device that will stay in the uterus until removed and must be inserted by a doctor. Insertion and removal will costs about $500. Some IUD's can be left in place for up to 10 years. The IUD prevents fertilization of the egg by producing a sterile inflammatory response that kills sperm. Some IUD's release progesterone and prevent implantation. A small string hangs out of the uterus into the vagina. A woman has to be able to feel this string in order to know that the IUD is in place. A woman should check the IUD string after every menstrual period. IUD's are 97% effective.

Due to some problems, the use of IUD's decreased in the United States during the 80's and 90's while the devices remained popular worldwide. The FDA recently approved the use of Mirena. Mirena is 99% effective and can be kept in place for up to 5 years if checked yearly by a doctor.

Possible Side Effects
- Expulsion of the IUD (rare)
- Menstrual Problems

Diaphragm

The diaphragm is a barrier method of birth control. A diaphragm is a round dome shaped rubber device that fits inside of the vagina and covers the cervical opening. A woman has to be specially fitted for a diaphragm by a doctor and this device must be placed in the vagina prior to sexual activity. To increase the effectiveness of the diaphragm Spermicide should be used. After a change in weight or child birth a woman should visit her doctor to get refitted for her diaphragm.

Common Complaints
- Inconvenient
- Skin irritation from Spermicide

The Birth Control Patch

Ortho-Evra is the first birth control patch to be introduced on the market. The patch is a thin square that can be worn in one of four places on the body. Ortho-Evra works by releasing small amounts of estrogen and progesterone into your system. The patch is 99% effect. Ortho-Evra became available for prescription in April of 2002.

Possible Side Effects
- Headaches
- Menstrual Cramps

Common Complaint
- May slip off when wet

The TODAY Sponge

The Today Sponge was introduced in the United States in 1983. It soon became one of the leading selling over the counter birth control methods on the market. The sponge can be inserted into the vagina. It has the spermicide Nononxonol-9. It is effective for up to 24 hours. The sponge is popular because it allow spontaneity and there are no hormones involved but the effectiveness rate ranges between 84-91%. The Today Sponge is currently available in Canada. As of publication time, it was due to be re-introduced into the American market.

Possible Side Effects
• Burning, itching or vaginal irritation for the woman (or her partner) if one has an allergy to nonoxynol-9.

Emergency Birth Control
Preven, or the "morning after pill" can be used within 72 hours of having unprotected sex. It is 98% effective. Preven is a form of emergency contraception and should not be used as a regular birth control method. Preven is the first FDA approved emergency contraception. Preven stops or delays ovulation after sexual intercourse has taken place. Preven is only available by prescription.

Common Complaints

• Drug stores sometimes do not have the product in stock, thus reducing the effectiveness if a woman has to wait several days for the drug to arrive.

• Woman has to visit or contact a doctor immediately in order to get the drug prescribed.

Chapter 10- Web Resources

ABORTION

The National Abortion Federation
www.prochoice.org
The National Abortion Federations mission is to keep abortion safe and legal. Their web site features abortion facts, information on finding an abortion provider and links to relevant web sites.

Abortion Clinics On-Line
www.gynpages.com
Abortion Clinics On-Line is a directory service of abortion providers.

Planned Parenthood –Abortion
www.plannedparenthood.org/ABORTION/
A part of the Planned Parenthood web site, the abortion section includes factual information about the abortion procedure. Site also includes a Q&A section that features answers to common questions about abortion.

National Network of Abortion Funds
www.nnaf.org
The National Network of Abortion Funds provides support to local abortion funds, aids in the creation of new abortion funds and helps women who are having financial difficulties finding the funds for an abortion.

Mifeprex- Medical Abortion Pill/RU-486
www.earlyoptionpill.com
Official web site for the early option abortion pill. Site includes answers to commonly asked questions about Mifeprex and information about the history of the early option pill.

ADOPTION

National Adoption Information Clearinghouse
http://naic.acf.hhs.gov
The National Adoption Information Clearinghouse is a resource with a wealth of information on adoption. The Clearinghouse is a service of Children's Bureau, Administration on Children, Youth and Families, Administration for Children and Families, Department of Health and Human Services.

Bright Futures Adoption Center
http://www.bright-futures.org
Bright Futures Adoption Center, Inc. is a non-profit adoption agency that educates and guides birth parents and adoptive parents through the adoption process.

Independent Adoption Center
www.adoptionhelp.org
Founded in 1982, The Independent Adoption Center is a non-profit organization that strives to make adoption a viable option for women seeking to place their children up for adoption.

Insight-Open Adoption Resources and Support
www.r2press.com
Brenda Romanchik explains the process of open adoption on her web site. She is also the author of several helpful adoption pamphlets that educate birth parents on the adoption process.

American Association of Open Adoption
www.openadoption.org
In depth site with extensive information about open adoption. Their purpose is to give you the best information available about adoption.

American Adoption Congress
www.americanadoptioncongress.org
The American Adoption Congress is composed of individuals, families and organizations committed to adoption reform. They represent people whose lives are touched by adoption. Their web site includes valuable information about the adoption process.

Adoption.Com-Where Families Come Together
www.adoption.com
Adoption.com is an on-line adoption resource site. Site includes information for the birth mother and prospective adoptive parents.

Lifetime Adoption Facilitation Center
www.lifetimeadoption.com
Lifetime Adoption provides birth parents with assistance in finding prospective adoptive families. Services are free to birth mothers.

ANTI-ABANDONMENT/SAFE HAVEN

A Safe Haven For Newborns
www.asafehavenfornewborns.com
A Safe Haven For Newborns has a listing of state by state Safe-Haven laws and other information about Safe Haven legislation.

Project Cuddle
www.projectcuddle.org
The Project Cuddle web site provides a 24 hour hotline for women considering abandoning their infants. Site also features information on how Project Cuddle can assist pregnant women who are in desperate situations.

BABY DIAPERS

Huggies
www.huggies.com

Luvs
www.luvs.com

Pampers
www.pampers.com

EXPECTING MOTHERS

Storknet- Pregnancy and Parenting On-Line Community
www.storknet.com
The Storknet site features nutrition information, a baby name database, message boards and a wealth of pregnancy related information.

Babyzone- Pregnancy, Parenting and Family Planning
www.babyzone.com
Babyzone is an on-line community for the expecting parent. Site features a wealth of pregnancy related articles, links, and resources.

Pregnancy Today- Pregnancy and Baby Related Resources for Parents By Parents
www.pregnancytoday.com
The Pregnancy Today site features a daily pregnancy calendar, diaries, personal web pages and various other pregnancy and parenting related resources.

American Baby-Your Partner In Parenting
www.americanbaby.com
The American Baby site features expert advice, a pregnancy calendar, and various other parenting and pregnancy related information. You can also subscribe to American Baby magazine for free via the web site.

Pregnancy Week By Week
www.pregnancyguideonline.com
Pregnancy Week by Week is a comprehensive site that features fetal developmental information about each week of pregnancy. Site also includes information about how mom to be will be feeling during her pregnancy and reviews of pregnancy books.

BREASTFEEDING

Breastfeeding.com-Information, Support and Attitude
www.breastfeeding.com
This breastfeeding web site includes a breastfeeding Q&A section, expert advice, video clips, and instructions on how to express breast milk.

La Leche League
www.lalecheleague.org
The La Leche league web site provides a wealth of breastfeeding information and a directory of local La Leche League groups.

CHILD CARE

National Child Care Information Center
www.nccic.org
The National Child Care Information Center is a national resource that ensures all children and families have access to high-quality comprehensive services.

The Original Babysitting Connection
www.babysittingconnection.com
The Original Babysitting Connection is an on-line resource that let parents search for child care providers in their area.

EMERGENCY CONTRACEPTION

Back Up Your Birth Control
www.backupyourbirthcontrol.org
This on-line campaign strives to educate women about emergency contraception. Site includes facts and informative information about emergency contraception.

Preven
www.preven.com
Preven is the Is the first FDA-approved product for emergency contraception.

GOVERNMENT RESOURCES

Women, Infant and Children Program (WIC)
www.fns.usda.gov/wic
WIC is a USDA program designed to provide nutritious food supplements and education to at risk pregnant women and their children.

Food Stamp Program
www.fns.usda.gov/fsp
The Food Stamp Program provides benefits to low income people so that they can purchase food to improve their diet.

The Administration for Children and Families
www.acf.dhhs.gov
This web site provides information on Administration for Children and Families programs including Welfare and Low Income Assistance, Child Care, Child Support, and other programs.

US Department of Health and Human Services
www.hhs.gov
The US Department of Health and Human Services web site provides links to agencies that fall under the Department of Health and Human Services, including Medicaid.

INFANT FORMULAS

Carnation Good Start
www.verybestbaby.com
The Carnation web site includes information about Carnations infant formula. Carnation also has a free magazine that expecting parents can subscribe to.

Enfamil
www.enfamil.com
The Enfamil web site features product information and child development information.

Similac
www.welcomeadditions.com
The Similac web site features product information and child development information.

MATERNITY LEAVE

Family and Medical Leave Act
www.dol.gov/esa/whd/fmla/
This site includes the 1993 text of the act, regulations, compliance guides, forms and related information regarding the act.

Facts About Pregnancy Discrimination
www.eeoc.gov/facts/fs-preg.html
The EEOC provides information about the Pregnancy Discrimination Act and a brief overview of a pregnant woman's rights and her employers responsibilities.

MATERNITY SHELTERS AND CRISIS SUPPORT

Lifecall
www.lifecall.org/shelters.html
The Lifecall web site features a state by state listing of maternity shelters

Children of the Night
www.childrenofthenight.org
Children of the Night is a not for profit organization dedicated to helping children between the ages of 11 and 17 who find themselves in the world of prostitution. They provide shelter and educational programs to help children in need.

Covenant House
www.covenanthouse.org
Covenant House is a private organization that provides food, shelter and clothing to homeless and runaway youths. In addition to providing shelter, they provide services in education, health care, and vocational training.

Pregnancy Center Listings
www.pregnancycenters.org
Web site features state by state listings for Pregnancy Centers (formerly known as Crisis Pregnancy Centers).

Birthright
www.birthright.org
Birthright provides guidance and assistance for women facing unplanned pregnancies. Birthright helps women find alternatives to abortion.

PARENTING SUPPORT

One Young Parent
www.oneyoungparent.com
One Young Parent is a support network for teen parents and their families.

Girl Mom
www.girlmom.com
Girl Mom is a web site for young mothers and aims to support young mothers of every kind.

Making Lemonade- Single Parent Support Group
www.makinglemonade.com
Making Lemonade is an on-line support system for the single parent. Web site features include forums, classified section, single parenting dating information and much more.

Parents Without Partners
www.parentswithoutpartners.org
This is the official web site for the organization devoted to the interests of single parents.

SAFER SEX AND BIRTH CONTROL

Depo-Provera
www.depo-provera.com
Commonly known as the "Birth Control Shot", Depo-Provera is birth control you only have to worry about 4 times a year.

Epigee-Birth Control Guide
www.epigee.org/guide
The Epigee birth control guide features information about contraception currently available.

Reality-The Female Condom
www.femalehealth.com
The Female Health Company is the company that makes the Reality Female Condom, the first female condom on the market.

Today Sponge
www.todaysponge.us
As of publication time, the Today Sponge was set to be re-introduced into the American market.

Mirena
www.mirena-us.com
Mirena is a long lasting birth control device that is placed in the uterus.

Ortho Evra
www.orthoevra.com
Ortho Evra is the first birth control patch on the market.

SEXUAL EDUCATION AND SUPPORT

Planned Parenthood
www.plannedparenthood.org
Plannedparenthood.org is the official web site for the worlds largest reproductive health care organization. The web site features a wealth of information on a variety of topics.

Its Your Sex Life
www.itsyoursexlife.com
It's Your Sex Life aims to raise sexual awareness. Site features information on pregnancy, contraception, and sexually transmitted diseases.

Coalition For Positive Sexuality

www.positive.org

The goal of the Coalition For Positive Sexuality is to teach people positively about sexual education

Teenwire

www.teenwire.com

Teenwire provides sexuality and relationship information sponsored by The Planned Parenthood Federation of America.

TEEN PREGNANCY AND PREVENTION

National Campaign To End Teen Pregnancy

www.teenpregnancy.org

The goal of the National Campaign to Prevent Teen Pregnancy is to reduce the rate of teen pregnancy by one-third between 1996 and 2005. Site features resources, articles, quizzes, and tips for teens and parents.

Chapter 11- Phone Numbers

AMT Children of Hope Foundation
Infant Emergency Pick-Up Hotline
1-877-796-4673

Lifetime Adoptions Birth Mother Hotline
1-800-923-6784

Carnation Good Start Infant Formula
1-800-248-8107

Child Abuse Hotline
800-4-A-CHILD (800-422-4453)

Child Care Aware
1-800-424-2246

Crisis Pregnancy Hotline
1-800-662-2678

Covenant House 9-Line
1-800-999-999

Children Of The Night
1-800-551-1331

Emergency Contraception Hotline
1-888-not-2late

Enfamil Infant Formula
1-800-baby-123

Food Stamp Hotline
1-800-221-5689

Helpline
1-888-467-8466

Mifeprex-Early Option Hotline
1-877-432-7596

National Adoption Information Clearinghouse
1-888-251-0075

National Domestic Violence Hotline
1-800-799-SAFE (800-799-7233)

National Network of Abortion Funds
413-559-5645

Planned Parenthood
1-800-230-plan

Project Cuddle 24-Hour Hotline
1-888-628-3353

Birth Right Pregnancy Hotline
1-800-550-4900

Similac
1-800-227-5767

STD Info Line
1-800-227-8922

Youth Crisis Hotline
1-800-448-4663

WIC Hotline
1-800-342-5942

Chapter 12-Related Reading

ABORTION

Abortion-A Positive Decision
Author Patricia Lunneborg
Bergin & Garvey; ISBN: 0897892437; (May 1992)

The Abortion Resource Handbook
Author K. Kaufmann
Fireside, ISBN 0684830760 (July 1997)

Behind Every Choice Is a Story
Author Gloria Feldt
University of North Texas Press, ISBN 1574411586; (January 2003)

The Choices We Made: Twenty Five Women and Me Speak Out About Abortion
Authors Angela Bonavoglia (Editor), Gloria Steinem
Publisher: Four Walls Eight Windows; ISBN: 1568581882; (March 30, 2001)

Our Choices, Our Lives: Unapologetic Writings on Abortion
Author Krista Jacob
Publisher: Iuniverse Star, ISBN: 0595298230; (January 2004)

A Solitary Sorrow : Finding Healing & Wholeness After Abortion
Authors Teri K. Reisser, Paul, Md. Reisser, pa Reisser
Harold Shaw Pub; ISBN: 0877887748; (January 2000)

ADOPTION

The Adoption Resource Book
Author Lois Gilman (Preface)
Harper Reference; ISBN: 0062733613; 4th edition (November 1998)

The Complete Idiot's Guide to Adoption (Complete Idiot's Guides)
Authors Christine A. Adamec, Chris Adamec, Chris Adamac, William Pierce
MacMillan Distribution; ISBN: 0028621085; (January 1998)

The Essential Adoption Handbook
Author Colleen Alexander-Roberts
Taylor Pub; ISBN: 0878338403; (December 1993)

Children of Open Adoption and Their Families
Author Kathleen Silber, Patricia Martinez Dorner
Corona Pub; ISBN: 0931722780; (February 1990)

Dear Birth Mother
Authors Kathleen Silber, Phylis Speedlin
Corona Pub; ISBN: 0931722209; 3rd edition (December 1998)

The Open Adoption Experience: A Complete Guide for Adoptive and Birth Families--From Making the Decision Through the Child's Growing Years
Authors Lois Ruskai Melina, Sharon Kaplan Roszia (Contributor)
Harper Perennial; ISBN: 0060969571; (November 1993)

SINGLE PARENTING

The Single Parent Resource
Authors Brook Noel, Arthur C. Klein, Art Klein (Contributor)
Champion Pr Ltd; ISBN: 1891400444; 1 edition (May 1998)

The Single Mother's Survival Guide
Authors Patrice Karst
Crossing Pr; ISBN: 1580910637; (March 2000)

The Single Mother's Book : A Practical Guide to Managing Your Children, Career, Home, Finances, and Everything Else
Author Joan Anderson
Peachtree Publishers; ISBN: 0934601844; (July 1990)

The Complete Single Mother
Authors Andrea Engber, Leah Klungness
Adams Business Media; ISBN: 1580623026; 2nd edition (March 1, 2000)

On Our Own : Unmarried Motherhood in America
Author Melissa Ludtke
University of California Press; ISBN: 0520218302; (March 1999)

PREGNANCY

I Wish I Had Waited
Author Sylvia Willis Lett
Letts Dream Big Publishing; ISBN: 0-9761829-0-4; (Sept 2004)
http://www.lettsdreambigpublishing.com

A Child Is Born
Author Lennart Nilsson
DTP; ISBN: 0440506913; Revised edition (May 1, 1986)

The Girlfriends Guide To Pregnancy
Author Vicki Iovine
Pocket Books; ISBN: 0671524313; (October 1995)

The Pregnancy Book
Authors Williams, Md. Sears, Martha Sears, William Sears, Linda H. Holt
Little Brown & Co (Pap); ISBN: 0316779148; (June 1997)

While Waiting
Authors George E. Verrilli, Anne Marie Mueser, Marie Mueser (Contributor)

Griffin Trade Paperback; ISBN: 0312187750; 2nd Rev edition (June 1998)

The Mother of All Pregnancy Books
Author Ann Douglas
Hungry Minds, Inc; ISBN: 0764565168; 1st edition (January 1, 2002)

You Look Too Young to Be a Mom: Teen Mothers Speak Out on Love, Learning, and Success
Author Deborah Davis
Perigee Books, ISBN 0399529764 (April 2004)

SEXUAL EDUCATION AND REPRODUCTIVE HEALTH

Sex, Boys & You: Be Your Own Best Girlfriend
Author Joni Arredia
Perc Publishing, ISBN 0965320324 ; (September 1998)

Smart Sex
Authors Jessica Vitkus, Marjorie Ingall, Jessica Weeks
Pocket Books, ISBN: 0671019104; (March 1998)

The Go Ask Alice Book of Answers: A Guide to Good Physical, Sexual, and Emotional Health
Author Columbia University's Health Education Program
Owl Books, ISBN: 0805055703; (September 1998)

This Book Is About Sex
Authors Tucker Shaw, Flona Gibb, Fiona Gibb
Puffin Books, ISBN: 0141310197; (October 2000)

DISCUSSION QUESTIONS

Questions for women currently pregnant

1. If this pregnancy was unplanned, how do you plan to prevent future unplanned pregnancies?

2. If your boyfriend asked you to participate in a DNA paternity test how would you feel? Would you allow the test to be performed on you and the baby? How would this affect your relationship?

3. If you plan to raise your child, do you think being a parent will force you to alter any of your future goals?

4. Who has helped you the most with your unplanned pregnancy?

5. Will you have to change your living arrangements due to your impending birth if you plan to raise the child?

Exercises for women currently pregnant

1. Keep a journal to document your pregnancy.

2. Make a list of the things that you need to purchase for your upcoming delivery. Itemize your purchases into the following categories—Must Have, Optional, Can Wait.

3. Write a letter to your unborn child. In the letter detail your feelings about your pregnancy and your expectations for the birth and motherhood.

4. Write a birth plan. In this plan, detail how the events of your child's birth will unfold. Plan for who will watch your other children if you have any, how you will get to the hospital and

every detail. Discuss with your doctor before hand if you plan to use pain medication during your labor.

Activities

1. Plan a "The baby's not here yet!" party. Invite your good friends. Rent your favorite movies and encourage your guests to bring your favorite food dishes so that you won't have to cook.

2. Take a trip to the store. Price items that you will need to purchase on a monthly basis (such as diapers, formula, etc.) Prepare a monthly budget for these items.

3. Plan for child care. Visit day care centers and home providers and determine which setting you will utilize. Prior to visiting each setting, write a list of questions to ask the providers about their facility or home day care operation. Write a list of the pro's and con's of each day care provider.

General discussion questions

1. If you were faced with an unplanned pregnancy what would you do?

2. Who would be the first person that you would first confide in about your unplanned pregnancy? Why?

3. Young women shared their stories of unplanned pregnancies in this book. Which stories stood out the most in your memory?

4. What section of this book did you find the most helpful?

5. Have you ever had a friend or family member confide in you about their unplanned pregnancy?

Abortion

1. Do you think abortion should remain legal in this country?

2. Do you think that if abortion was illegal that women would still pursue the procedure?

3. What are your feelings about parental consent and/or notification laws? Are these laws necessary?

4. What are your feelings about mandatory waiting periods?

5. Do you think that it is difficult for women to obtain accurate information about abortion?

Adoption

1. If you are considering adoption, would you prefer an open or closed adoption? Why?

2. If you are considering a closed adoption, would you want to leave open the possibility for your child to be able to contact you when they reach adulthood? Would you want the adoption to be completely confidential?

3. Did you ever consider kinship adoption? If so, which family member would you approach about adopting your child?

4. How would you resolve a situation if the child's father did not want to take full custody of the child, yet he objected to the child being placed for adoption?

5. If you ever considered keeping the baby or having an abortion, what made you decide on adoption as an option?

About The Author

Dorrie Williams-Wheeler is an author, educator and designer. She completed her Masters of Science of Education degree from Southern Illinois University. She is a popular teen author. Her fiction titles *Be My Sorority Sister-Under Pressure* and *Sparkledoll Always Into Something-2004 Edition* have both garnered awards and critical acclaim. She is also the author of the non-fiction book *The Unplanned Pregnancy Handbook*, a similar pregnancy book written for an older audience.

As a freelance writer Dorrie has written for Teenwire.com and the Teen section at Bellaonline.com. She is also the founder of the popular 80's site imissthe80s.com and the urban entertainment site thabiz.com. You can visit Dorrie on the web at www.dorriewilliamswheeler.com or www.dorrie.info.

The mother of two resides in Virginia Beach, Virginia with her husband.

Be sure to visit The Unplanned Pregnancy Book for Teens and College Students on the web at www.unplannedpregnancybook.com!

About The Publisher

Sparkledoll Productions releases fiction and non-fiction titles for the mature teen/college age female audience. Visit us on the web at www.sparkledoll.com.

REFERENCES

Brewer Sforza, Gail and Janice Presser Green. *Right From The Start.* Emmaus: Rodale Press, 1981.

Erickson, Kristen. "Benefits of Breastfeeding." *Today's Pregnancy* Birth Options Issue 2001: 7.

Fields, Denise, and Alan Fields. *Baby Bargains: Secrets to Saving 20% to 50% on Baby Furniture, Equipment, Clothes, Toys, Maternity Wear and Much, Much More!.* New York: Windsor Peak Press, 2001.

Glasier A (1997). Emergency postcoital contraception. New England Journal of Medicine, 337(15): 1058–1064.

Hamburg Copland, Jill. "Baby Bucks Money & More-Safe and Secure." *Babytalk*
    March 2002: 64.

Huggins, Kathleen, R.N., M.S. *Nursing The First Two Months.* The Harvard Common Press, 1991.

Kuzemchak, Sally ; Jones, Sarah. "Birth Control Choices-A Roundup of What's
    New and What Works Best Post-Baby." American Baby May 2002: 61-65.

Link, David, M.D., Editor. *American Baby Guide To Parenting.* New York:
    Gallery Book, 1989.

Philadelphia Department of Public Health. *Healthy Foods, Healthy Baby.*
    Philadelphia: Office of Maternal and Child Health. 1998.

Robinson, Bryan. "Delaware v. Grossberg and Peterson Grossberg To Serve

Two-and-Half Years; Peterson Receives Two-Year Sentence."
Court TV
     Trials. 09071998. Court TV. 01052002.

          <http://www.courttv.com/trials/grossberg/070998.html.>

Rosen, Peg. "Beyond Baby Blues." <u>American Baby</u> May 2002: 95-100.

Saving Babies Together. *Eating For Two.* Wilkes-Barre: March of
Dimes Birth Defects Foundation, 1998.

Spock, Benjamin,M.D., and Michael B. Rothenberg, M.D. *Dr. Spock's
Baby and*
     Child Care. New York: Penguin Books, 1992.

Virginia Department of Health. *Why Every Woman Needs Folic Acid.*
Richmond: 2001.

<u>Web References</u>

<u>Abortion.</u> Planned Parenthood of America. 14 August 2004.
          <http://<u>www.plannedparenthood.org/</u>ABORTION/>.

<u>Abortion</u>-What To Think About. Web MD. 13 August 2004.
          <<u>http://my.webmd.com/hw/womens_conditions/tw2458.asp</u> >.

<u>About Depo-Provera-How It Works.</u> Depo-Provera. 22 May 2004.
          < http://www.depo-provera.com/howitworks.asp>.

<u>About GE 4D Ultrasound.</u> GE 4D Ultrasound. 3 August 2004.
          <http://www.gehealthcare.com/rad/us/4d/about.html>

<u>ACLU Reproductive Rights: Mandatory Waiting Periods Before
Abortions.</u>   American Civil Liberties Union.   27
June 2004.
      <http://www.aclu.org/issues/reproduct/waiting_periods.html>.

<u>American School of Corresondence-General Facts.</u> American School. 21
August 2004.

<http://www.americanschoolofcorr.com>.

An Adoption Glossary. Bright Futures Adoption Center. 10 December 2004.
<http://www.brightfutures.org/birthfamilies/adoptionglossary.htm >.

Choices for an Abortion. Web MD. 17 May 2004.
<http://my.webmd.com/hw/womens_conditions/tw9202.asp >.

Court TV On-Line New Jersey vs. Drexler. Court TV On-Line. 5 April 2002.
<http://www.courttv.com/trials/drexler/>.

Dilation and Evacuation (D&E) For Abortion. Web MD. 11, Agust 2004
<http://my.webmd.com/hw/inflammatory_bowel/tw2462.as >

DNA Paternity Testing-FAQ. DNA Diagnostic Center. 18 August 2004.
<http://www.dnacenter.com/faq.html >.

DNA Paternity Test-FAQ. Swabtest. 18 August 2004.
<http://www.swabtest.com/faqs.php>.

Family Medical Leave Act. Department of Labor. 2 November 2003.
< http://www.dol.gov/esa/whd/fmla/ >.

Food Stamp Program. U.S. Department of Agriculture. July 2004.
<http://www.fns.usda.gov/fsp/>.

Frequently Asked Questions-Is Depo-Provera a Good Choice For Most Women?
Depo-Provera Contraception Injection. 17 June 2004.
<http://www.depo-provera.com>.

Frequently Asked Questions About DNA Paternity Testing. Genelex. 18 August 2004.
<http://www.genelex.com/paternitytesting/paternityfaq.html>.

GED. Prometrics GED Home. 22 August 2004.
<http://www.prometric.com/GED/default.htm >.

Government Issues New RU-486 Warning. FOX NEWS. 16 November 2004.
< http://www.foxnews.com/story/0,2933,138756,00.html >.

Housing Choice Vouchers. Department of Housing. 17 August 2004.
<http://www.hud.gov/offices/pih/programs/hcv/index.cfm>.

How Can Paternity Be Established? Illinois Child Support Enforcement. July 2004.
< http://www.ilchildsupport.com/paternity_cs.html >.

How Mifeprex Works. Mifeprex. 2 April 2002.
<http://www.mifeprex.com/how.php3>.

Induced Abortion U.S. The Alan Guttmacher Institute. 3 August 2004.
< http://www.agi-usa.org/pubs/fb_induced_abortion.html>.

Introduction to Adoption. National Adoption Information Clearing House. 13 July
2004. < http://naic.acf.hhs.gov/parents/index.cfm >.

Just Another Girl On The I.R.T. All Movie Guide. 14 August 2004.
<http://ww.allmovie.com>.

Prenatal Peek-Services. Prenatal Peek Site. 8 August 2004.
<http://www.prenatalpeek.com/index.htm>.

Prom Mom Admits Killing Newborn. CNN.Com. 28 April 2002.
<http://www.cnn.com/US/9808/20/prom.birth.02/ >.

Reproductive Waiting Periods. ACLU. March 2004.
<http://archive.aclu.org/issues/reproduct/waiting_periods.html>.

RH Sensitization During Pregnancy. Web MD. August 12 2004.
<http://my.webmd.com/hw/being_pregnant/hw135945.asp>.

Routine Prenatal Tests. Kids Health For Parents. 2 April 2002.

<http://kidshealth.org/parent/system/medical/prenatal_tests_p4.html>.

Safe Haven Laws. A Safe Haven For Babies. 17 August 2004. <http://asafehavenfornewborns.com/laws.html>.

Safe Haven Laws for Abandoned Babies Cause Problems. Fox News. 25 August 2004. <http://www.foxnews.com/story/0%2C2933%2C80645%2C00.html>.

Teen Sex and Pregnancy. The Alan Guttmacher Institute. 23 May 2004. <http://www.agi-usa.org/pubs/fb_teen_sex.html>.

Tenant Based Housing. Department of Public Housing. 14 August 2004. <http://www.hud.gov/offices/pih/programs/hcv/tenant.cfm>.

Today Sponge-An Overview. Today Sponge US. 29 August 2004. <http://www.todaysponge.us/overview.htm>

What Is Mirena? Mirena USA. 22 April 2004. <http://www.mirena-us.com/consumer/whatisframe.html>.

WIC At A Glance. U.S. Department of Agriculture. 12 April 2003. <http://www.fns.usda.gov/wic/>.

Yale School of Nursing finds that teen parents and their babies both do better when high schools offer child care. Yale School of Nursing . 27 August 2004. <http://www.nursing.yale.edu/news/daycare.htm>.

Vacuum Aspiration for Abortion Surgery Overview. Web MD. 13 August 2004. <http://my.webmd.com/hw/womens_conditions/tw1078.asp>

Dorrie Williams-Wheeler